CONTENTS

——

INTRODUCTION

—

'The health of a population depends on the way in which political actions condition the milieu and create those circumstances which favour self reliance, autonomy and dignity for all, particularly the weaker.'
Ivan Illich, *Medical Nemesis*, 1977.

Some people look at the world as it is and ask why. I look at the world as it could be and ask why not? I believe that governments do what they believe they can get away with; as a result Britain has one of the worst records in Europe on environmental pollution and health. It seems to me that most of our health problems are political, rather than technological. The biggest improvement in our health this century has come, not from drugs or the medical profession, but from clean water, decent sanitation, better housing, improved transportation and working conditions, better education and more information.

Information is power. The quality of any decisions you make about your health care depend upon the quality of your information. Pasteur recanted germ 'theory' just before he died. The human 'climate', he said, made a difference, so that in a healthy body 'germs' would not proliferate well. Nevertheless he had set a trend in medical thinking which is still adhered to even though, I believe, it is wrong.

Natural health care is about observing, respecting and using correctly the natural laws of the universe. Nature is a whole and no one part can equal the whole. Taking a few chemicals from a plant and throwing the rest away because they appear to have no therapeutic value denies a basic principle of nature and provokes iatrogenic side effects (effects that are produced only through the treatment administered). Two out of every five people on drugs suffer from side effects, in many instances more serious than the problem which the drugs are being used to treat.

Holistic medicine does not treat symptoms but takes the total picture into account. Its scope includes the emotional, mental, spiritual, social and environmental aspects of a person's life, not simply the physicalities they present. Herbal medicine assists the forces of nature and respects nature's laws. I hope that our passion for chemistry is palling. Our greed for the short-term 'easy' fix has turned forests into wastelands, agricultural land into deserts and seas into cesspits, as well as provoking a situation in the so-called developed nations of the world where two out of every three people die of cancer or heart disease, both degenerative diseases which are largely preventable. If you eliminate junk food, exposure to chemicals at work, smoking, excessive drinking, housing and hobbies full of environmental hazards, and undue stress, and add the alchemy of plants, you have the most superb preventative system in the world and give the planet a chance to begin slowly to recover from the crippling things we have done to it.

Plants offer their healing not just to us but to the earth. Plants breathe in what we breathe out. Through the nitrogen–carbon cycle of chemical change animal waste is transformed by plants into food and medicine. Repair, nurture, heal. This is the heritage we should leave to our children, because with all of these things comes hope, perhaps the most important medicine of all.

Use the information in this book to keep yourself and your family well. The first chapter is concerned with health maintenance. I am a great believer in nipping disease in the bud. In parts of China doctors are paid only when their patients are well and payment is stopped if they became ill. This truly preventative approach would revolutionize current health systems in the Western world!

Read chapter 2 with care before attempting to make any formulations. Knowing is one thing; doing quite another. The Resources Directory at the back of the book lists suppliers who will prove invaluable in this instance. The list of contraindicated herbs (pages 63–71) must always be checked before making a formulation.

Chapter 3 gives you basic routines to keep yourself healthy; this seems to me as sensible as putting your car in for a regular service. Chapter 4 deals with the hazards of living in a modern world and how to protect yourself and your family from them. Thousands of years ago the most famous physician of all, Hippocrates, knew that fresh air and water, and appropriate exercise, were central to good health and that the study of the patient's environment was a vital part of correct diagnosis. Indeed, with breathtaking simplicity his Hippocratic School suggested that environmental and emotional factors were often the only conditions that needed correcting if a patient was to get well.

The second half of the book is an easy A-to-Z of common ailments. Having said that, I rarely name a disease: I prefer to acknowledge conditions, by looking at a person as a whole, rather than treating a sore arm or a bloated stomach. However, for ease of reference and general understanding I have used terms such as 'arthritis', while keeping my approach as holistic as possible given the constraints of a reference-book format and the fact that I am not personally acquainted with the patient.

If in doubt, don't diagnose yourself. Even the most understanding GP only makes an accurate diagnosis 50% of the time, if he has no access to pathology laboratories. Alternative medicine also offers many accurate methods of diagnosis, some of which are discussed here. I, for example, am an iridologist and a vega tester and have found these alternative methods of diagnosis extremely useful and generally accurate. The whereabouts of similar practitioners are described in the Resources Directory. If in doubt about any aspects of your health, seek the advice of a qualified herbal practitioner. The British Herbal Practitioners Association – an umbrella group of most of the herbal schools in the UK – will be happy to supply you with the name of a practitioner. It is part of the European Practitioners Association, listed in the Resources Directory.

Consider a general check-up before you encounter any health problems. By the time many people come to see me, they have often been seen by more than one specialist, and perhaps undergone surgery before being rejected as 'incurable'. Too often, conventional practitioners are only concerned with a narrow biomedical approach to the treatment of disease which results in fragmented treatment that is both ineffective and inflationary. We need to change the direction of current medical thinking with a quiet revolution. I believe we will not be able to maintain, let alone increase, our well-being until we make profound changes to our value systems and social organization. Meanwhile, I hold my candle and hope it will eventually kindle enough unlit ones to create an illuminating blaze.

Glimmers of light are beginning to dawn. The United States has stopped jailing its herbalists, although my own teacher, Richard Schulze, a leading American herbalist, has been persecuted so severely by the FDA over many years that he has now been forced to close his practice. His teacher, Dr Christopher, went to jail many times in defence of his profession. Germany now sends its hard-pressed executives to recuperate in naturopathic clinics (where disease is treated by natural means only). Herbal medicine is now available in most French and some Italian pharmacies and the Czech Republic and Hungary boast some of the best health spas in Europe. Witch doctors hold conferences and are considered perfectly respectable in Zimbabwe. China continues to revere its 'barefoot doctors' as among the most skilful diagnosticians in its medical network. The World Health Organisation (WHO) is now positively encouraging Third World countries to continue to use the herbal medicines they have used for centuries. This is a perfectly sensible move, not simply in economic terms but in philosophical and empirical terms. Ancient Indians in Peru surveyed canals down steep mountain slopes at such precise angles, and following such sophis-ticated scientific principles, that we would have to use satellites and laser beams to match them. Certain native North American tribes planted crops along the top of curiously shaped mounds that apparently raised the temperature several degrees and gave them a week or two of extra growing time in the autumn. Why should traditional cultures be any less discerning about their health?

I hope that we continue to forge on with multidimensional approaches and emerge with a standard of health that has hitherto been only a dream.

CHAPTER 1
HEALTH MAINTENANCE

———

Doctors are trained not to prevent disease through a healthy lifestyle and good diet but to treat with drugs and surgery. A recent American investigation showed that the average doctor in the United States received less than three hours of training in nutrition, for example, during four full years at medical school (British doctors may receive six or eight hours). Given their paucity of training, they can hardly be blamed for not relaying the emerging truths of modern nutritional research to their patients. Instead, doctors are trained to: 'wait until deformed and mentally retarded babies are born, then give them loving attention; wait until heart attacks come, then if the patient is still alive, give him or her the best care possible; wait until mental disease strikes and give considerate treatment; wait until alcoholism strikes, then turn to the task of rehabilitation; wait until cancer growth becomes apparent, then try to cut it out or burn it out with suitable radiation' – in the view of Roger J. Williams in his *Nutrition Against Disease* (Bantam Books, 1973).

The lowest life expectancy in the world, often only about 30 years, is held by the Inuit, Laplanders, Greenlanders and the Kurgi tribes in Russia. The common denominator? They are the populations with the highest animal flesh consumption in the world. Interestingly, other people living in harsh conditions but who, for cultural or economic reasons, are only able to eat small amounts of animal flesh (if any) have some of the highest life expectancies in the world: they include the Russian Caucasians, the Yucatán Indians, the East Indian Todas and the Pakistani Hunza-kuts. Average life expectancy among these people ranges from 90 to 100 years. The Vilcambas, who live in the Andes in South America, the Abkhasians, who live on the edge of the Black Sea, and the Hunzas, who live in the Himalayas in the northern part of Pakistan, hold the record for the longest lifespans in the world. The factor that linked all three tribes together? They were, in spite of being in completely different parts of the planet, almost totally vegetarian. In addition to longevity, these tribes had full, active healthy lives throughout their years and showed very few signs of the degenerative diseases that afflict the elderly in the Western world.

In the West, far from getting healthier, people are succumbing to chronic degenerative diseases including high blood pressure, heart disease, cancer, diabetes, circulatory problems, arthritis, obesity and mental disorders. They are subject to stress and environmental pollution, they over-eat and under-exercise.

In the US, life expectancy for men and women of all ages is falling and infant mortality is on the increase. In Britain, the number of babies born congenitally malformed or who grow up educationally subnormal has been rising steadily since the 1940s. Britain has the highest death rate from heart disease in the world, as well as the worst infant mortality figures in Europe. After the age of 45, our life expectancy is among the lowest of any developed country.

The cost of allopathic – the opposite of homeopathic; that is, rather than treating like with like, treating disease by 'inducing' disease of another kind – health care in the West is escalating. The British National Health Service (NHS) stumbles from one financial crisis to another and the rocketing cost of health care in the United States is a major political issue. Iatrogenic disease, that is disease caused by medical examination or treatment, is actually on the increase. Every year people die following operations which are not strictly necessary; in the UK one in six hospital beds is currently used by those suffering from adverse reactions to chemical drugs.

The majority of the British population 100 years ago was underfed, underweight and short of protein, vitamins and minerals. Now we eat 100 lb (45 kg) of sugar and 100 lb (45 kg) of fat per head per year, and two-thirds of the energy in our food comes from sugar, alcohol and fats. Three-quarters of our food is processed, much of it poor and empty of vitamins, minerals, starch, dietary fibre and protein. Many of the convenience foods we eat have chemicals added whose long-term affects are unknown and cumulative. If we add to this the dangers of air laden with industrial pollutants or cigarette smoke, and a less-than-perfect water system, we are clearly in trouble.

The pharmaceutical industry is one of the biggest in the world. Next is the agricultural and food-processing business. In economic terms, those foods which are the best commodities are ones which take up little space, travel well and do not rot. Sugar is concentrated, pure, cheap, does not go off, tastes nice, is uniform and easy to make (as well as transport and pack), so it is considered the best commodity of all. It is a relatively cheap, stable bulking agent found in the majority of packaged food.

The most profitable fats are the most unhealthy ones. Those found in vegetable seeds, nuts, fresh green vegetables, some fruits and fresh fish are unstable, tend to go rancid quickly and are therefore unpopular as far as food processing is concerned. Saturated fats are solid, stable at room temperature, and travel well and cheaply.

As a nation, we are also highly addicted to salt which was once used as a preservative but for which – since our discovery of freezing, cook-chill methods and accelerated drying – we now have little use.

There is a collusion between what is currently good for health and what is good for business and the consumer comes out the loser. Potatoes boiled in their jackets or baked in their skin are undoubtedly healthy, particularly if they are organic, but potatoes which are turned into snacks become unhealthy and expensive. Yet it makes economic sense to turn potatoes into such snacks before we buy them, because the whole process uses technology, machinery, advertising, packaging and, of course, people, hence the massive profitability of some sections of the food industry. But there is light at the end of the tunnel. There are a few supermarkets and food processors in Britain who are actively trying to make their products more healthy, and use less fat, sugar and salt, additives and preservatives in their manufacture.

Most of us have only vague notions of what a well-balanced diet is all about. The majority of us suffer from sub-clinical deficiencies which, if left unchecked, cause a slow but inevitable physical decline. Of the 28,000 people surveyed by the Health and Nutrition Examination Survey between 1971 and 1974 in America, half the women had calcium deficiencies, iron deficiency was common among people of every race, income group and cultural background, and 60% of the people who took part in the survey overall had at least one symptom of malnutrition.

If we are to seriously improve the health of the nation we must begin with our children before they are even conceived and continue during pregnancy, at birth and in their developing years. We pass on our genetic blueprints to our children. If you come from a family with a history of allergies, hay fever or asthma, it is much more likely that your children will suffer from the same problem. If they have had to wear glasses or have a mouth full of fillings in spite of a reasonable diet, the chances are that you, your parents, and even your grandparents have all been lacking in adequate nutrition. It is possible to change this predictable pattern by looking at your own state of health well before you attempt to conceive.

If you have a particular health problem and you are planning a family for some time in the future, resolve now to put all your energies into eliminating it or at least elevating your overall health as far as you can. I advise my patients to allow at least a year to prepare for a really healthy conception. It is advisable to seek professional help in order to do this, but if you have or have had in the past an unhealthy lifestyle (perhaps involving a highly processed diet, smoking, heavy drinking, drugs, obesity or lack of exercise) it is also possible to do something about this yourself. You will need to find ways of tackling malnutrition at a cellular level, remembering that it takes almost 100,000 different chemicals to keep your body working properly and that all these chemicals work synergistically. So far, nutritional science has isolated less than 60 of these in vitamins, minerals, amino acids and other co-factors. But they are all there in natural, uncontaminated food.

The greatest and most durable gift you can ever pass on to your children is a clear understanding of the philosophy behind your own diet and lifestyle. You need to be persistent and make it enjoyable so that good health and all that its maintenance entails become second nature to your children.

Our nutritional needs are as different and as individual as our fingerprints and vary according to our lifestyle and life stage. They are affected by stress, illness, puberty, pregnancy and lactation, the menopause, old age and environmental factors. What is less clearly understood is that structural and enzymic differences, which are partially determined by genetics, decide how you absorb any nutrients. For example, it is possible that you may be continually urinating away nutrients simply because your renal threshold is low, or you may have insufficient intestinal bacteria to ensure the absorption or manufacture of a certain nutrient.

Who is right and who can you believe? I have been in clinical practice for 15 years and seldom see people who come to me simply for a preventative check-up. I tend to deal with those who are seriously ill. In my clinical experience, the advice I am about to give you has the greatest potential for quickly rebuilding health, preventing disease and maintaining excellent health – and it is about diet. It works because I have tried it with thousands and thousands of patients over the years and seen the results. Their bodies have been my laboratory.

TEN PRINCIPLES FOR SUPERB NUTRITION

1 FOR OPTIMUM NUTRITION EAT LIBERALLY FROM THE THREE BASIC FOOD GROUPS: VEGETABLES; FRUITS; SEEDS, NUTS AND GRAINS.

SEEDS, NUTS AND GRAINS

These should be eaten mostly raw and sprouted, but they also contain all the important nutrients essential for healthy growth, as well as for prevention of disease, when cooked.

Sprouted seeds are particularly valuable because they increase their nutritional content phenomenally once they germinate. If you sprouted oats, by the time a seed had put forth two tiny green leaves, it would have increased its vitamin B content by 2,000%. The vitamin C content in soya beans rockets five times once sprouted. Indeed you could live off sprouted grains and seeds alone and remain entirely healthy (and wealthy as they are so cheap to grow). They contain a synergistic balance of amino acids, natural sugars and fatty acids, as well as vitamins and minerals, essential unsaturated fatty acids and lecithin. They also contain pacifarins, an antibiotic-resistant factor that increases natural immunity, as well as auxones, natural precursors of vitamins that help to rejuvenate the body's cells and prevent premature ageing. They are also bulky, which is essential for the normal function of the digestive tract and the prevention of all sorts of digestive diseases including diverticulitis, appendicitis and cancer of the colon.

Grains which do need to be cooked are better pre-soaked and low heated. To do this simply fill a wide-necked thermos flask with one-third grains and cover with two-thirds of freshly boiled water. Leave the jar standing overnight with the stopper in and the next morning when you open it you will find the grains have popped open and are plump, juicy and ready to eat. Yet they are still live and if you tried to plant them in the garden they would sprout (this would not be possible had they been boiled).

ESSENE BREAD

The best flours are chickpea, millet, spelt, quinoa, soya and rice. The healthiest bread to eat is Essene bread pioneered by the ancient Essenes thousands of years ago: its basic ingredient is whole wheat or rye grains pre-soaked for 15 hours and then sprouted for two or three days. You should then grind them as finely as possible in a food processor adding a touch of oil to form a ball and place on a bread board sprinkled with wheatgerm to stop the dough from sticking. Roll it into a thin sheet with a rolling pin dusted with wheatgerm or press it out with your fingers on a flat tray as thinly as possible without breaking it. Leave the bread on top of a radiator or on a warm stove or even in a cool oven with the pilot light turned on for between six and twelve hours, turning over halfway through with a wide spatula. It has a sweet nutty flavour and a delicious biscuity texture. There are also commercially produced breads made from sprouted seeds, which are available in health-food shops and are dense, sweet and delicious.

The next healthiest bread after those from sprouted seeds is sour dough bread because during the natural souring process there is an enzymic action on the grain producing valuable lactic acid which makes it easily assimilable.

Naturally beans (such as kidney, haricot, mung and flageolet), peas and lentils can be cooked and flavoured as desired.

VEGETABLES

Wherever possible, vegetables should be eaten raw in the form of salads, baked, steamed or stir fried in a little cold-pressed olive oil. Eating them raw or juiced is preferable to cooking them. (Cooking destroys many vitamins in vegetables, particularly the water-soluble ones B and C.)

Steaming is one of the healthiest (and easiest) ways to cook vegetables: steamers are widely available in kitchenware shops and department stores, or use a sieve over a saucepan of boiling water (keep the lid on – and protect your hands by picking up the sieve with a pot holder as the handle will be hot).

Many people do not realize that vegetables are also good sources of protein. Potato is 11% protein, pumpkin 15% and cabbage 22%. As a substitute for salt when cooking vegetables use savoury kitchen herbs, cayenne, seaweeds, soya sauce and generous amounts of garlic and onions. Try to use organically grown vegetables which are in season, whenever possible.

FRUITS

Fruits are a cleansing food. Fruit juice, once assimilated by the stomach, will cleanse the blood stream within minutes of being drunk. Again fruits should be organically grown and in season as far as possible and they are excellent sources of vitamins, minerals and enzymes. Dried fruits are perfectly acceptable as long as they are unsulphured and organically grown. Don't go for the ones which are rolled in white glucose powder or are suspiciously shiny. This means they have been coated with paraffin wax. Think about chewing a candle and that should put you off buying them! Fruits and fruit juices are best eaten for breakfast in the morning or as a snack late at night if you are still hungry.

*

Each one of these three food groups should supply the bulk of one of your three meals. Ideally fruit for breakfast; seeds, nuts or grains for lunch; and vegetables for dinner, although this order can be changed.

2 EAT RAW LIVING FOODS AS FAR AS POSSIBLE

As much as 75% of your diet should be raw. This is not as daunting as it sounds if you drink several large glasses of freshly juiced fruits or vegetables daily and make a large salad one of your main meals (home-made sauerkraut and pickles count as raw food). Enzymes, vitamins and minerals are easily destroyed by cooking which also changes the biochemical structure of amino acids and fatty acids, making them only partially digestible.

Food eaten raw prevents digestive leucocytosis; that is, the number of white cells in the bloodstream does not increase. Processed and cooked foods induce white cell mobilization, so it is advisable to always begin any cooked meal with something raw. The problem with leucocytosis is that each time white blood cells flood into the intestines to combat cooked food the rest of the body is left unguarded: this strains the immune system. Raw foods liberate the white blood cells for other more important tasks, stopping this constant defensive action. A 100% raw food diet, while ideal, is impractical, particularly in a cold or temperate climate. However, if I am treating somebody who is very ill, I do ask them to go on raw juices and raw foods, sometimes for many months, in order to accelerate their healing.

THE POTENCY OF RAW FOOD

Dr Max Bircher-Benner, a Swiss nutritionist and visionary, understood the potency of raw food. 'Mangez vivant!', he told his patients, meaning 'Eat living food'. He had no objections to eating meat, as long as it was uncooked and in its entirety of blood, fat, bones, entrails, skin and flesh – in other words, exactly the way a lion eats prey in the wilderness. He understood that as soon as any food was processed in some way, it altered the state of the whole-food energy and produced ill health.

A more acceptable way to enjoy raw foods is to eat plants. We have the ability to protect the delicate enzymes in such food as it passes through our digestive tracts so that about 70% reach the colon intact. By binding with oxygen, enzymes enhance the activity of our intestinal flora. Too much oxygen in the digestive tract encourages putrefaction and intestinal toxaemia; fermentation has been linked with all sorts of degenerative diseases including digestive cancers. Foods which are rich in enzymes include freshly sprouted seeds, grains and pulses, pawpaw, pineapples, and fermented foods such as sauerkraut and rejuvelac, the water collected off soaked wheat before it is sprouted.

RED MEAT AND DISEASE

The highest level of cancer, shared between men and women, in the Western world is colonic or rectal cancer, which accounts for 60% of all cancers. Red meat is heavily implicated in this type of cancer. The probable reason for this is that, when the cholesterol in meat is worked on by bacteria in the colon, by-products are created that are powerful carcinogens. When beef is barbecued, the fat that splatters into the fire is changed by the heat into benzopyrene, a potent carcinogen. This chemical rises in the smoke and coats the surface of the steak; when the meat is chewed and swallowed, it is smeared against the bowel wall during the course of the digestive process.

A diet high in red meat increases the risk of breast cancer. This is because cows, lambs and pigs bred for slaughter are fed hormones and antibiotics, the residues of which remain in active form in the meat. Women who eat animal fat create high levels of the hormones oestrogen and prolactin, and these stimulate the growth of breast tissue, as well as the uterine lining and other tissues. As a result, women who eat red meat have higher rates of tumours and cancers of both the breast and uterus.

All forms of concentrated protein (this includes chicken, fish and eggs, as well as meat) injure the kidney filters, contributing to kidney failure, as well as leaching calcium from the bones, leading to osteoporosis.

Meat also contributes to chronic inflammatory conditions, of both the bronchial tubes and joints. This may be the result of the constant assault on the immune system by foreign animal products inherent in all meat and dairy products. *The Lancet* has reported that animal protein and animal fat actually aggravate arthritis symptoms, and every single one of the patients in the reported study, when put on a pure vegan diet, noticed a significant improvement very quickly. Of asthmatics placed on a vegan diet, 90% were able to reduce and some were even able to entirely discontinue their medication. There is mounting evidence that that a high-fibre, low-fat plant-based diet is of central importance in both the prevention and treatment of a broad range of diseases. It has been conservatively estimated that vegans have only 40% of the national cancer rate and have a lifespan six years greater than average.

The BSE Issue

Bovine spongiform encephalopathy, or mad cow disease, is a highly infectious and currently an incurable disease which attacks the brain and nervous system of cattle. Scrapie, a similar disease found in sheep, has been recognized for 200 years; the nearest human equivalent is Creutzfeldt–Jakob disease (CJD). The exact origin of BSE is not known. It is, however, neither a virus nor a bacteria – indeed nobody knows what it is – and it seems to have broken the most basic rules of biology.

BSE has been epidemic in the British cattle industry for the last 10 years and by 1994 had been identified in 150,000 animals and cases had been acknowledged in over half of all the cattle herds in Britain. It has not yet been proven that BSE can be transmitted to humans but regular eaters of veal and other beef products are 13 times more likely to die of CJD than those who don't eat such products. There is a real prospect that large numbers of people will die from CJD in the next century; some scientists now feel that CJD and BSE are one and the same thing.

After four years of Government reassurances that BSE could not possibly infect other species, tests carried out in February 1990 proved the exact opposite: BSE was transmitted to mice through food. In May 1990 a domestic cat died from spongiform encephalopathy and by July (after the death of 52 more cats) the Government acknowledged that it was being contracted through eating pet food. By 1991 BSE was transmitted experimentally to seven out of eight species of mammal, including pigs and marmoset monkeys, in four cases through food. CJD claimed the lives of two dairy farmers who had tended herds with BSE-infected cattle.

By 1994 the Government was having to admit that cows could and did pass on BSE to their calves. In *Nature* of 25 April a team from Oxford University added further evidence to the growing concern that humans are particularly at risk from BSE. Professor Richard Lacey, the first scientist to alert Britain to the risks of BSE, said: 'The research reveals a freak characteristic in Prp proteins which are shared by both humans and cows and of which the prion is a variant. It suggests a strong evolutionary relationship between cattle and humans and supports the case for easily transferred disease from one to the other, in particular CJD v. I have always believed that CJD originated in cattle and this new variant of it has been naturally selected to withstand extreme heat, to survive in a wide variety of hosts and to have extreme potency. The new research reveals that humans are likely to be highly susceptible to BSE–CJD. It is inexcusable that the Government should be claiming beef is safe when most of the evidence is pointing in the opposite direction.'

Juliet Gellatley, the founder and director of Viva!, pointed out: 'Cow manure carries the BSE agent and yet it is still spread on fields where cattle graze and from which silage is cut. There is transfer from cow to cow through the shared eating of placentas and there is some cross-contamination from injections. The Government's refusal to accept that there is an internal transmission when the evidence is overwhelming reveals its sole concern is to keep a lid on this crisis in defiance of the truth.'

After almost 10 years, expert knowledge on BSE–CJD is almost non-existent. Professor Lacey's worst-case scenario is that CJD could be responsible for 500,000 deaths annually for many years. Sir John Pattison, the chair of SEAC, a government body formed to advise on spongiform encephalopathy advisory matters, admits that Professor Lacey could be correct. The SEAC report acknowledged that it is impossible to measure the risk because no one knows the strength of the species barrier, that is, how easily the disease could be passed from cattle to humans. Also, although it is clear that high levels of the BSE agent can cause infection, no one yet knows what prolonged exposure to low levels will do. The Government claims that the period of greatest risk to meat eaters in Britain was between 1986 and 1989, before the specified offal ban was introduced and brains, spinal cords, tonsils and other offal were supposedly removed from the food chain.

Until 1986, such items could be found in cheap beef products such as sausages, burgers, stocks and pies. After introducing the ban, the Government made no effort to police it. Subsequent slaughterhouse checks revealed that in almost 50% of cases the controls were ignored. Policing of the system is carried out by the Government-appointed quango, the Meat Hygiene Service. There has been widespread flouting of herd controls, with farmers obtaining false certificates declaring their herds are BSE free. More than 75,000 calves from infected herds were shipped abroad prior to 1996, so that BSE is probably widespread in continental Europe.

In 1989 the Government banned the use of feed containing the remains of other animals for cows but it is still in use for pigs and sheep. Bonemeal, blood and offal are still used on fields as fertilizer and the Government's own scientists have expressed fears that this practice may have infected our rivers and water supply. The Government has now banned the use of bonemeal on commercial fields but continues to allow it for use in domestic gardens.

It is not known whether gelatine poses any dangers. Milk and dairy products are supposed to be free from white blood cells, believed to be the carrying agents for BSE, and, in theory, should be safe for human consumption. But cows catch mastitis and are supposed not to be milked when affected; and this depends on farmers observing the rules, noticing an outbreak when it starts and being certain that it is cured before milking again.

The simplest and safest answer to BSE and CJD is to stop eating animals until such time as the Government supplies accurate, reliable and truthful information about the epidemic.

FISH

Fish and fish oils are often described as particularly helpful to a healthy diet. Today, however, rivers and oceans are often heavily contaminated with pesticides and toxic chemical residues, with the result that it is almost impossible to find fish from unpolluted waters. Fish are at the top of an extremely long food chain because bigger fish eat little fish; as a result of this exponential progression, large fish have dangerously high concentrations of pesticides, insecticides and other toxic chemicals, as well as detergents, industrial effluents, oil spillage, harbour dredgings, human and animal sewage, and ships' garbage. In view of all this, fish have been found to contain toxins known to be carcinogenic, and to cause kidney failure, nerve damage and birth defects.

The fish themselves display high rates of cancer. Pollutants, such as polychlorinated biphenyls (PCBs), DDT and dioxin, concentrate in the muscle tissue of fish and it has been estimated that eating a 1 lb (450 g) fish from Lake Ontario is the same as drinking 1.5 million quarts (1.7 million litres) of that polluted water. More than 80% of the fish taken from lakes and rivers in New York State, Ohio and Michigan showed cancerous tumours of the skin and liver visible to the eye. Carcinogenic hydrocarbons were found in fish in the rivers of Maryland, in the Nile, and in rivers in Florida, and there are increasingly alarming reports of carcinogenic residues in fish taken from the Mediterranean and Baltic seas.

Shellfish

Pollutants of the water become particularly heavily concentrated in those creatures that live at the bottom of the ocean, river or lake where the chemicals fall. Oysters, clams and mussels have all been found with excessive levels of pollutants and, as filter feeders, they eliminate contaminants through their faecal matter. As humans usually prefer to eat clams and oysters whole they munch not only the toxins concentrated in the tissue but also that trapped in faecal matter left in the intestinal tract. In 1984, mussels in California were found to have lead contamination 150 times greater than the maximum said to be fit for human consumption. Shellfish are capable of carrying toxic levels of lead, cadmium, arsenic and other heavy metals. Raw shellfish carry dangerous microbes and toxins and, since the introduction of raw fish in increasingly popular Japanese restaurants in the Western world, infections from parasitic worms have increased.

Mercury Poisoning

Poisoning from mercury results in nerve paralysis. It is becoming increasingly common among fish eaters. Large predatory fish such as halibut, tuna, swordfish, shark and marlin are particularly predisposed to mercury poisoning. Mutagenic PCBs tend to gravitate to the flesh of trout, catfish, bass, carp, bluefish and mackerel – and mackerel are particularly fond of feeding off human sewage. The Irish Sea is the most radioactive sea in the world, and contamination from nuclear-power plants affects fish.

Trade Secrets

In 1978 the Thames Water Authority discovered hermaphrodite fish in the river Lee, which supplies drinking water to London. The effects on rats of drinking sewage-contaminated water was studied for eight years, until the results were deemed 'unsuitable for publication'. The Ministry of Agriculture, Fisheries and Food carried out some of the research in 1990. They found that rainbow trout and carp mutate when exposed to low levels of sewage and oestrogen hormones from contraceptive pills, but the results were only revealed two years later in the *Foundation for Water Research Journal*. New research is funded by private industry, but heavily cloaked in commercial confidentiality clauses. Companies need permits to release toxic effluents into the sewage systems and inspectors monitor the discharges. Their reports are available, but it is a criminal offence to disclose information from the records without the consent of the water company, making it illegal to pass on or publicize the findings.

In the United States food inspection reports are available to the public through the Freedom of Information Act. In Britain, records of hygiene and veterinary inspections by the Ministry of Agriculture, Fisheries and Food at all British abattoirs are secret because they refer to individual plants and must remain confidential. Only food exported to the United States and therefore scrutinized by the US Food and Drug Administration (FDA) has publicly available hygiene inspection reports.

Fish Oils

Over the last few years these have been lauded as protective against clogged arteries and heart attacks. But this needs careful thought. The liver of the fish, like the liver of any other vertebrate, is the central organ for processing chemicals, so the chemicals which accumulate in the flesh of the fish are particularly concentrated in its liver. Fish oils are extracted from the liver of the fish. They actually decrease the body's ability to coagulate to stop bleeding. While the rate of heart attacks among Inuits who eat largely fish is low, they suffer from the world's highest rate of haemorrhagic strokes, nosebleeds and epilepsy. Inuits also have the highest osteoporosis rate in the world.

Fish oils have recently been found to increase the length of a normal pregnancy; an overly long pregnancy increases a baby's weight, which may escalate the risk of birth accidents, the necessity for caesareans and maternal deaths. Late-birth rates in the Faroe Islands are among the highest in the world and death rates in late pregnancy are also high. Fish oil contributes to gall bladder disease and it is high in cholesterol. Far from being brain food, a lot of fish is so high in mercury that it actually poisons the brain and nerve cells.

Farmed Fish

The flesh of farmed salmon is made to look appetizingly pink by a dye mixed with its feed. Farmed fish are kept in cages and, therefore, can breed diseases. Trout are particularly prone. Fish farmers use Dichlorvos to get rid of sea lice in salmon. The US Environmental Protection Agency have classified this as a potential carcinogen and it is listed by the British Government as one of the most dangerous chemicals that can enter the waterways. Yet, until 1992, its use was condoned.

Both the Dutch and German Governments have warned people not to eat flatfish caught in the North Sea because they consider them too diseased and contaminated with a whole range of conditions, including liver disease, skin lesions, viral diseases and genetic abnormalities. If you want to eat fish:

- Buy from deeper, cleaner, oceans than the North Sea. Ask your fishmonger where it came from.
- Cook fish well.
- Treat what you catch yourself cautiously. Consider getting its purity confirmed by your local environmental health officer.
- Don't buy frozen fish whose origins are not labelled, or mixtures of fish in pre-prepared food such as fishfingers.
- Campaign for cleaner waterways and seas. Don't be disappointed if you hit blank walls: when Friends of the Earth asked for information about the quantity

and toxicity of sewage sludge supplied to farmers, their request was turned down by the Severn Trent Water Authority who said: 'The names of individual farmers, their addresses, grid references of private farm land, etc., form part of the Register, but are clearly data of a personal nature we could not provide to others.'

The good news is that by significantly reducing your consumption of all meats, fish, dairy products and eggs, you will have an even lower heart disease rate than the famous Inuits and should have an extremely low risk of osteoporosis.

EGGS

Eggs contain no fibre and are high in fat and cholesterol. They contain eight times more cholesterol than the equivalent weight of beef and if you have ever dropped an egg on to a lino floor you will know that it bonds as well as wallpaper paste. The walls of Venice were built of eggs and mud more than 500 years ago and they are still standing! This should give you some idea of just how difficult eggs are to digest.

Between one and five colourants are fed to chickens to give a richer colour to the egg yolk; one of these, canthaxanthin, was banned by the Ministry of Agriculture Fisheries and Food for direct human consumption. Chickens are also fed arsenic to kill parasites and stimulate growth, and naturally this comes out in the eggs they ovulate. Besides this, eggs are rich in sulphur which strains the kidneys and the liver. Chickens eat their own and each others' droppings which means they are continually recycling their own infections through their and their fellow chickens' bodies. If you want to continue to eat eggs, buy free range, or preferably organic (now available in larger supermarkets). But they really aren't necessary – I use soya cream in my baking: one level tablespoon takes the place of an egg nicely.

CHICKENS

In the USA 37% of chickens carry salmonella, a figure that has been constant for the last 10 years. A lesser percentage of beef and pork is contaminated in this way, too. Having been killed, once opened the inside of the carcasses are sprayed with chlorinated water to reduce the bacterial count but the current method of screening a chicken for salmonella relies on visual signs of infection and even schoolchildren know that you can't see bacteria with the naked eye. If you eat chicken in the belief that it is low fat, you should know that 2½oz (75g) of boiled chicken contains as much fat as 2½oz (75g) of hamburger.

I trained as a professional chef and spent some of my youth in private houses and hotels in Europe and America, happily ladling on gallons of cream, seasoning and alcohol in true old-fashioned *haute cuisine* style. At one time, I worked in a steak house grilling hundreds of steaks every night. My conversion to whole food and vegetarianism did not come as a Saul-on-the-road-to-Damascus experience. It began gently with my training as a medical herbalist but started to rage, full flood, when I was confronted by a burgeoning number of patients who were digging their own graves with their knives and forks through ignorance. It became obvious to me that many of the illnesses they brought me, chronic degenerative conditions – various cancers, sclerotic illness, diabetes, hypoglycaemia, allergies and arthritic and rheumatic diseases – were induced by apathy about health care on a general level, but especially by ignorance of diet. So my own philosophical veganism springs from my passion for preventative medicine. To paraphrase Lucan's *Pharsalia*, 'Observe moderation, keep the end in view, follow the laws of nature'. So buy your food wisely, cook simply if you have to cook at all, and cook well. Take some trouble to learn about the nutrients different foods contain so you can protect your own and your family's health and, above all, enjoy your new way of eating.

3 EAT NATURALLY AS FAR AS POSSIBLE

Ideally your food should be whole, unprocessed and unrefined, cultivated on fertile soil without the use of inorganic fertilizers, pesticides or insecticides. In other words it should have nothing removed and nothing added. White bread, for example, has over 20 nutrients removed and only four added. The apocryphal story of the packet being healthier than the cornflakes is in fact true.

4 EAT POISON-FREE FOODS

Organically grown vegetables and fruits contain more vitamins and minerals than those grown with the aid of chemicals. Not many additives have been tested for safety simply because of the enormous numbers involved. The few that have, have been tested in the scientific double-blind trial manner, one at a time, on healthy, well-fed animals. In the real world, of course, we are more likely to be eating different additives at once and their composition could be further altered by cooking methods. In Britain, we allow more additives and have weaker controls on them than any other major industrialized country.

More than 1 billion lb (453 million kg) of chemicals are added to food in the USA every year. By our late teens most of us have eaten 8 oz (225 g) of coal-tar dyes and as adults we eat 5 lb (2.3 kg) of additives each year. A growing number of us are becoming intensely susceptible to them. Dr John Hunter, a specialist in food allergy with extensive clinical practice dealing with migraine, asthma, rhinitis, urticaria, eczema, Crohn's disease and other digestive disorders, categorically states that one-fifth of his patients react to food additives. The snack market is growing by 10% per year and its labels read like a chemistry set. Words like 'permitted antioxidant' cover a multitude of sins. Two of the antioxidants which are widely used to prevent fats and oils from going rancid, butylated hydroxyanisole (BHA) and butylated hydroxytoluene (BHT), accumulate in body fat. They are present in virtually all manufactured foods containing any form of fat. BHA upsets the proper functioning of the intestinal muscles. BHT is believed to increase levels of fat and cholesterol in the blood, to induce birth abnormalities, stunted growth and baldness, liver and kidney damage and noticeable changes in brain chemistry. The UK Standards Committee have recommended twice that neither antioxidant be used in food, yet it is still widely used in many of the convenience foods that contain fats.

1 billion gallons (4.5 billion litres) of liquid pesticide are used yearly on Britain's farms. The London Food Commission's report *Food Adulteration and How to Beat It* states that of the major 426 chemicals used legally in 3,009 brands of pesticides and fertilizers, 164 have been implicated in causing cancer, genetic mutations, irritant reactions and reproductive problems, ranging from impotence to birth defects. Friends of the Earth state that a single lettuce can be sprayed as many as 46 times, onions 15, and potatoes 8.

If you simply can't find organic food, there are now non-toxic sprays available in health-food shops which remove chemicals from the skins of fruits and vegetables (see Resource Directory).

In the real world you are bound to come across foods that are poisoned by chemicals which will inevitably get into your system to some degree. Read the advice on page 90 about detoxing on heavy metals.

One of the diagnostic methods I use is vega testing. This, basically, reads the flow of electrical energy in the body through acupuncture points to test organ dysfunction, as the result of either fungal, viral or bacterial infection, or toxicity from various sources including heavy metals and industrial chemicals such as insecticides or pesticides. Instead of excreting toxins, the body tends to store them – particularly in the liver and in fat cells – and they remain trapped for many years causing slow, insidious but relentless damage to the body. I have never seen a patient who does not show poisoning from additives, preservatives, insecticides and pesticides.

5 AVOID DAIRY PRODUCTS

I am certain that the milk of any species was designed for one purpose only: to feed its young. Humans are the only creatures on earth who regularly drink the milk designed for another species. The enzymes we need to break down and digest milk are renin and lactose, but by the age of four most of us have lost the ability to digest lactose simply because we can no longer synthesize the digestive enzyme lactase. This lactose intolerance results in diarrhoea, flatulence and stomach cramps. If your ancestors are from Africa, particularly East Africa, China, the Philippines, New Guinea or Asia, or if you are a native American, Australian Aborigine or Inuit, your body is definitely not designed to digest milk properly. Some 20% of Caucasian children are also lactose intolerant.

To the list of problems naturally inherent in human consumption of milk designed for baby cows, I can append a whole host of unnatural ones.

- Cow's milk contains the accumulated pesticides that have been sprayed on the grain fed to cattle and often on the grass they eat.

- The female hormones given to cows increase milk production and body fats.
- The newly proposed use of the hormone bovine somatotrophin (BST) in milk will change its chemical composition and presents an uncertain danger to humans.
- Some milk has been shown to contain trace metals and radioactivity at higher levels than those permissible in drinking water.
- Some 20% of milk-producing cows in America are infected with the leukaemia virus which, because milk is pooled when collected, infects the whole milk supply. This cancer-inducing virus is resistant to being killed by pasteurization and has been recovered from supermarket supplies. Is it a coincidence that the highest rates of leukaemia are found in children aged three to 13 who consume the most milk products and dairy farmers who, as a profession, have the highest rate of leukaemia of any occupational group?

Cream will clog your arteries, contribute to weight gain and encourage elevated hormone levels that may foster cancerous growths. Cheese is a particularly concentrated and indigestible food. Yellow cheeses are soaked in chemical dyes and the condensed protein of cheese is responsible for many migraines. Most ice cream is a travesty of anything made with real cream. It is generally manufactured from cooked tallow, suet and lard, all of which is boiled out of offal and scraps from abattoirs. This is then preserved with enough additives to support a chemical factory (although manufacturers are not required by law to list additives). Yogurt, often praised as a health food, is as bad. If you are eating it for all that healthy lactobacilli, you should be aware that you need to eat 16 fl oz (500 ml) in one go to get even a fraction of an ounce intact and unattacked by digestive juices to reach your lower colon. Supermarket shelves are packed with fruited yogurts groaning with sugar, artificial flavours and colouring, and gelatine or vegetable gum thickeners. The list of non-yogurt ingredients in frozen 'yogurt' is worthy of a well-stocked chemical factory. If you are still hanging on to your low-fat cottage cheese, consider that it is thickened with calcium sulphate (plaster of Paris).

WHEY

Only 10% of the milk needed to make up cheese ends up as cheese. The remaining 90% is separated out into whey. This is so toxic that it cannot be poured into sewers (it is 200 times stronger a pollutant than residential sewage). If it is dumped into streams, it will leach out all the oxygen and kill fish. If it is put into land fills, there is a risk that it may seep into our water supplies so the agricultural industry sells it to food manufacturers who put it as a bulk ingredient into baked goods, ice cream, luncheon meats, imitation chocolate, soup mixes and beverages. Ovaltine, for example, contains more whey than any other ingredient except for sugar.

Read your labels. Try carob powder or syrup mixed into heated soya milk if you like a hot chocolate drink at night. Carob, made from grinding up St John's locust beans, makes a superb chocolate substitute but does not contain any caffeine. It is massively high in minerals and is rich in vitamin B as well as containing a little vitamin A. Go for the lighter powder which is untoasted and tastes creamier.

The alternative to dairy products is soya, oat or rice milk, which are freely available in health-food shops, or you can make your own nut milks. Simply blend a cup of shelled nuts with four cups of water in a liquidizer at high speed for a minute or so, decant into a glass jug and leave to sit in the fridge overnight. Strain through a piece of cheesecloth or a sieve the next morning and add honey or a touch of vanilla essence to taste. The remaining pulped nuts can be added to homemade soup or vegetable stews.

Whey can be used as a disinfectant and gargled but must not be swallowed.

COLD-PRESSED VEGETABLE OILS

Too much saturated fat clogs the arteries, which can lead to heart disease, strokes and even cancer. There is a lot of fat hidden in sausages, baked goods and dairy products. Saturated fat raises blood cholesterol and increases the risk of heart attacks. It is present in all dairy products and animal flesh but the only two vegetable sources are coconut and palm oil which are occasionally used in baked goods.

Unsaturated fats (mono- or polyunsaturated) are high in calories so will not help your weight but they do have good effects on blood fats: the more unsaturated fat in the bloodstream, the less room for saturated fats. Some of the more insidious residues from pesticides latch on to animal fats. In a recent governmental survey, one-third of all sausages sampled, half of 150 burgers sampled and half of 177 cheeses sampled were rife with pesticide residues.

Olive oil actually lowers your cholesterol levels by reducing the low-density lipoproteins (LDLs) which cause heart disease and increasing high-density lipoproteins (HDLs) which protect us from heart disease. Of course, olive oil is still high in calories so if you are trying to lose weight use it sparingly and do check that it is cold pressed, meaning unprocessed. Refined oils are treated with chemicals (including caustic soda) to remove fatty acids, then bleached and deodorized by heating at very high temperatures for up to 12 hours. This alters their chemical structure so much that they have no health benefits. Heating any oil up to a point where it is smoking distorts its chemical structure and encourages the proliferation of free radicals in the body, so deep frying is not a good idea. When I heat olive oil for stir frying I put a little hot water into the bottom of the pan first and wait for it to steam before adding the oil. This stops the oil from getting too hot.

Food manufacturers have now developed non-fat fats in order to cash in on the slimming market. Avoid them. They are fluffed up with cellulose, synthetic sweeteners and additives and are about as artificial and unhealthy as they can get.

While low-fat spreads contain about half the fat of butter or margarine plus water and a substance like gelatine to stick it all together, wouldn't it in the long run be better to avoid such travesties and settle, if you must, for a little pure organic butter and use it sparingly? Remember that the French, Spanish, Italians, Greeks, Turks and Portuguese wouldn't dream of smothering their bread with a layer of fat simply because the quality of their bread is so good they don't need to. If anything, they put a bowl of olive oil, perhaps with a little garlic or some fresh herbs chopped into it, on to the table in which to dip the bread. Insist on good bread and follow this healthy habit. I often use tahini diluted with lemon juice to pour over vegetables like potatoes instead of dotting them with butter.

BUTTER VERSUS MARGARINE

Which is best? In order to solidify liquid oil into something that you can spread on bread you have to harden it; this process is called hydrogenation. The process was invented in the 19th century by a Frenchman to make a cheap butter substitute for the French navy, and at that time margarine was rightly regarded as 'poor man's butter' with an inferior status. Somehow we have run away with the idea that it is a healthier product than butter and by 1981 margarine was outselling butter for the first time since the Second World War.

The majority of margarines today are made with a wide conglomerate of fats and oils including corn oil, coconut oil, palm oil, lard, sunflower, soya and fish oils. Anything cheap will do. Although fish and animal oils are now seldom used in margarines and most claim to be made of 100% pure vegetable oil, this doesn't mean that such a product is necessarily healthy. It could, in fact, be highly saturated. The process of pushing hydrogen gas through oil in order to solidify it converts it to a totally saturated fat. Margarine is close to plastic in terms of its molecular structure, in other words, it is a dead food. Try melting it in your hands and you will find it is impossible. This means it will not support any type of bacteria or fungus. Imagine then what it does inside your body. While it will certainly give you the same number of calories as butter, with the added bonus of beta carotene and annatto (as additional colouring) it often includes mono- and diglycerides and maltodextrin and it could clog your arteries. The study carried out by the Harvard Medical School on more than 85,000 women over eight years found that those eating margarine actually had an increased risk of coronary heart disease.

The oils used in margarine are refined so their essential fatty acids (EFAs) are damaged. In addition, solvents from petrol are added to produce a lighter taste, better clarity and colour. Bleach further removes EFAs, trace minerals and vitamins. If you heat this artificial substance, it further damages the EFAs and the resulting oxidation creates damaging free radicals in the body. These dramatically increase your need for vitamins and minerals.

During the process of hydrogenation itself, transfatty acids (TFAs) are produced which have a different molecular structure from anything found in human tissues and these, too, have a negative affect on our bodies' abilities to use

EFAs. TFAs appear to disrupt the body's use of cholesterol simply because our bodies cannot produce low-density compounds which carry cholesterol so the cells have to work harder to synthesize it, so raising levels of it in the blood.

When buying non-hydrogenated margarine make sure that there is nothing chemical added. Never use margarine for cooking or frying and look out for hydrogenated margarine in baked goods, crisps and snacks. Ensure you get plenty of EFAs from walnuts, evening primrose oil, flax seed (linseed) oil and beans and pulses.

HONEY AND MAPLE SYRUP

If using maple syrup make sure it is organic and if using honey make sure that it is natural, raw, unheated, unfiltered and unprocessed. Honey increases calcium retention in the system, prevents nutritional anaemia and is helpful for kidney and liver disorders, colds, poor circulation and complexion problems, as well as being rich in minerals. Many commercial honeys which are not labelled organic are made by bees being fed directly on white sugar, so avoid them. Maple syrup, because it is the sap extracted from trees, is not liable to overstress the pancreas, but both honey and maple syrup should be used in moderation and should be avoided altogether if you are prone to hypoglycaemia.

THE SPECIAL PROTECTIVE SUPERFOODS

Spirulina

This is one of the most concentrated nutritious foods on earth. It is a blue/green alga, which was the original photosynthetic source of life on earth, 3 billion years ago; it has nourished people in Central America and Africa for centuries. It is composed of soft mucopolysaccharides and has no hard cellulose in its cell walls. Its protein, therefore, is beautifully digested and assimilated in the human body. Spirulina has the highest protein of any natural food (65% or more), far more than animal and fish flesh (15–25%), soya beans (35%), eggs (12%), or whole milk (3%). And 95% of this protein is digestible. This is particularly important for those suffering from intestinal malabsorption (coeliacs, those affected by candida, Crohn's disease, mucous colitis and many people over 40 who have dwindling supplies of hydrochloric acid in their stomachs).

Life in the Fat Lane

Spirulina is only 5% fat, far lower than almost any other protein source. One tablespoon (10 g) has only 36 calories and virtually no cholesterol. So spirulina is a low-fat, low-calorie cholesterol-free source of protein. A large egg, by contrast, yields 300 mg of cholesterol and 80 calories but only has as much protein as one tablespoon of spirulina.

Colon Cleansing

Engevita nutritional yeast, chlorella and spirulina are the only forms of protein that are not mucoid forming in the intestines. Spirulina acts as a metabolic activator directly on the body's tissues at a cellular level, promoting increased activity to burn up mucus-forming substances (such as the wastes from meat, eggs and dairy products). Spirulina acts as an aggressive cleansing herb that empties toxins from the body tissues into the lymph and is a superb addition in both fasting and colon-cleansing programmes. 130, 452 | 615·321

Spirulina and Hypoglycaemia

The minimal amount of carbohydrate in spirulina, 15–25%, consists of two polysaccharides which are easily absorbed by the body with minimum insulin intervention. Spirulina supplies rapid energy without taxing the pancreas so it will not precipitate hypoglycaemia. Indeed, it is actively helpful for controlling the sweeping blood sugar curves which so debilitate hypoglycaemics and this is one more reason why it is so useful in a fast. It is also the richest source of vitamin B_{12} in food, higher than beef, liver, chlorella or sea vegetables, so it is highly recommended in a vegan diet. It actually reduces cholesterol, triglyceride and LDL levels. This may be partially due to its unusual and very high gammalinoleic acid (GLA) content. One tablespoon of spirulina provides 100 mg of GLA and dietary GLA helps heart conditions, PMT, obesity and arthritis.

Spirulina and Immunity

The unique colour in spirulina, phytocyanin, has been proved to stimulate the immune system and accelerate normal cell control functions, to prevent the degeneration of malignancies such as cancer and to inhibit its grown or reoccurrence. And the National Cancer Institute in America have found the glycolipids in spirulina to be remarkably active against the AIDS virus.

Spirulina encourages healthy lactobacilli by 327% over 100 days and increases the efficient absorption of vitamin B_1 inside the caecum, the part of the colon most prone to encourage the breeding of parasites, by 43%. Healthy lactobacilli mean better digestion and absorption, protect from infection and stimulate the immune system.

Spirulina and Anaemia

The iron in spirulina is twice as easily absorbed as the iron found in vegetables and meat and it is therefore highly recommended for people prone to anaemia. Spirulina was used to treat the 160,000 children suffering from radiation poisoning at Chernobyl. Remember that in addition to the toxic waste produced by nuclear-power plants we are all constantly exposed to radiation from the atmosphere, leaking microwave ovens, electrical power lines, X-ray machines, illuminated neon signs, clock faces, garage door openers and frequent flying. Spirulina also inhibits the growth of bacteria, yeast and fungi which is why it is so important as part of the candida-controlling programme, and to heal internal bacterial infections. A diet of 30% spirulina has been shown to radically decrease the toxicity of inorganic mercury and chemical anodynes, antibiotics and anti-cancer drugs which can cause acute nephrotoxicity (poisons in the kidneys).

Chlorella

Another of the blue-green algaes, this is second only to spirulina in its nutritional content. Its cell walls have to be artificially cracked to make the nutrients more available and increase its digestibility, so my first preference is always for spirulina over chlorella simply because any substance which has had to be artificially handled takes it one step further away from nature. Having said this, chlorella has some unique additions. Where spirulina is a multicell, spiral-shaped plant which grows on salty or brackish water, chlorella is a round, single-cell algae which grows on fresh water and it is unique in that it contains five times as much chlorophyll as spirulina. It is also different from spirulina in as much as it contains chlorella growth factor (CGF). In a study conducted by Dr Yoshio Yamagishi published in 1961, 50 10-year-old students given 2 g of chlorella daily for 112 days outstripped their control group in height and weight over this period of time. Chlorella's capacity to stimulate growth in the young is probably due to its nucleic acid content of RNA and DNA, which are important building blocks for life. RNA and DNA accelerate growth in the young and help repair damaged tissue in adults.

It has been suggested that the loss of energy and physical deterioration associated with ageing is due to the increasing breakdown of DNA and RNA, which are needed to keep the cells healthy. As we age (starting in our 20s) our natural production of RNA and DNA becomes sluggish. A diet rich in RNA and DNA foods produces more energy, and a more youthful appearance, and can alleviate long-standing problems such as arthritis, memory loss and depression.

The Importance of Chlorophyll

All plant life depends upon the sun. We depend upon those plants. Sunlight activates the green chlorophyll in plants to generate energy for them. Molecules of chlorophyll are constructed around magnesium and carry oxygen around the inside of plant cells which, in turn, creates energy for the plant. It is this stored energy in plants which we eat and absorb to sustain us. Plant energy is the primary energy of life because even carnivores eat animals which eat plants.

Our vitality depends upon a good supply of oxygen. Germs gravitate towards tissue which is oxygen deficient. Cancer tissues grow by a process which does not use oxygen. Whether taken internally by mouth or rectally by enema, chlorophyll inhibits the activities of protein-destroying bacteria and of those enzymes which make protein putrefy in the gut. It helps to make human saliva more alkaline, particularly helpful if you are eating carbohydrates. Chlorophyll can therefore be very helpful in the treatment of allergies and for malabsorption problems.

The Advantages of Taking Chlorophyll

Those of my patients prone to viruses such as flus and colds are generally either anaemic or smokers. Fewer haemoglobin molecules means reduced oxygen-carrying capacity for red blood cells. Smoking makes the haemoglobin of red blood cells bind with carbon monoxide, found in cigarette smoke. Whenever oxygen is wanting in our cells disease sets in. Both chlorophyll and haemoglobin molecules are capable of carrying oxygen to cells and in fact they are fairly similar in construction.

Many years of research have found that chlorophyll is not a chemical which is good for a specific disease but one which benefits the entire body by carrying oxygen to every cell. Consequently chlorophyll can help many different conditions including:

- sinusitis
- colds
- rhinitis
- respiratory infections
- colon problems including ulcerative colitis
- high blood pressure
- skin infections
- pancreatitis
- peptic ulcers
- gastritis
- mouth sores
- boils
- fatigue
- cancer
- septic wounds.

It increases resistance to X-rays.

Japanese researchers have found that the juice of any green plant inhibits chromosome damage which is one of the links in the chain of events leading to cancer.

All grasses contain fresh chlorophyll. Indeed there was a village in Austria during the Second World War which had all its food supplies commandeered by occupying troops. The population consequently lived off grasses. Amazingly, not only did they thrive but many of their more degenerative diseases began to heal completely. While you might blanch at the thought of eating grasses the good news is that other dark green vegetables like spinach, cabbage and nettles also contain large amounts of chlorophyll as, of course, does chlorella.

The CGF factor noted in chlorella is also present in wheat and barley grass. To obtain all its benefits it must be administered orally or as a rectal injection and it must be made freshly. Synthetic chlorophyll won't do and is in fact poisonous.

Barley and Wheat Grasses

Naturally, barley and wheat grasses can be sprouted but when grown in soil they are more potent nutritionally than the grains themselves, richly abundant with vitamins, minerals and chlorophyll; barley is twice as rich in protein as wheat.

Growing your own grass in order to eat it may sound exceedingly eccentric but the dividends are well worth it. When using wheat or barley grass juice for the first time it is a good idea to take it in very small quantities, perhaps only a tablespoon to begin with. Take enough to make you feel uncomfortable but not so much that you feel like vomiting it up again. Because both are such powerful cleansers due to their high enzyme contents they will start immediate reactions with toxins and mucus in the stomach, often causing distress. This feeling of nausea merely proves that they are needed and should be taken regularly. Drink a quarter of a lemon squeezed into a glass of water 30 minutes before drinking grass juice or, if you have an acid stomach, mint tea. Both methods will clean out mucus from the stomach and minimize discomfort.

Try and take any grass juice on an empty or nearly empty stomach. That way it is immediately absorbed. If you find in spite of all this that it is so potent you simply cannot swallow it it may be taken by rectal implant, in which case use a minimum of 4 fl oz (100 ml) working up to 8 fl oz (250 ml) daily. Raw grass juices can be used as a mouthwash. Remember chlorophyll will bring oxygen to the mouth and this is particularly helpful for anyone who has thrush or candida in their mouth or throat.

Purple Dulse, Kelp and Other Seaweed

Of all the seaweeds, dulse has the richest mineral concentration but I particularly like it because it tastes bland. I found many other types of seaweed, including kelp, taste rather fishy. All sea plants contain the minerals and trace minerals that are found in the oceans and the earth's crust and are easily assimilable.

All seaweeds are rich source of organic iodine, valuable in overcoming poor digestion and goitre, and in rebuilding and maintaining the function of all the glands. They are useful as an adaptogen in thyroid disease of any description.

Beetroot

Beets change inorganic raw elements into plant materials that are easy to assimilate. Beetroot is particularly famous for its blood-building ability. It is used in the treatment of cancer and is a superb liver and blood cleanser. Raw grated beets and their juices were once used to treat tuberculosis, obesity and gonorrhoea. The plant pigments in beets are particularly helpful to both cure and prevent radiation-induced cancers.

Dark Green Leafy Vegetables

All dark green leafy vegetables, especially spinach, are high in calcium, iron, vitamin K and, of course, chlorophyll. If you are juicing any dark green vegetables, use the juice in very small quantities as it is extremely potent – if you try to drink them by themselves, your mouth will soon tell you this is the case! The organic oxalic acid found in beet greens, Swiss chard, kale, turnip greens, broad-leafed sorrel and spinach, all in their raw state, is excellent for constipation. Once cooked, the oxalic acid can settle in the joints so if you are prone to gout or rheumatism don't eat these vegetables cooked.

In the 1950s the conservative British Ministry of Health and Public Service Laboratory admitted that spinach juice, cabbage juice, kale and parsley were far superior to milk for relieving excessive production of hydrochloric acid in the stomach.

Rosehips, Orange and Lemon Peels

These are some of the best sources of vitamin C and contain the whole vitamin C complex, including bioflavonoids, rutin, hesperidin, calcium and all the trace elements that are now known to be necessary in vitamin C assimilation. All citrus peels contain pectin, which removes heavy metals such as mercury and lead and even radioactive contamination like strontium-90 from the body. When you eat citrus fruit, always eat some of the white pith as it contains bioflavonoids.

Bioflavonoids

However, the bioflavonoids in the pith of all citrus fruit is highly active and unstable and easily destroyed by heat and exposure to the air.

Two of the bioflavonoids appear to have even better anti-inflammatory properties than cortisone while others, singularly or together, actively fight fungal, viral and bacterial infections. Quercitin is exceptionally active against viruses, particularly herpes. Rutin, famous for elasticizing arteries, also lifts depression, by altering brain-wave patterns and acts as a preventative against bruising. It is richly present in buckwheat. Nobiletin helps the body to get rid of heavy metals and the poisonous substances from car exhausts, and is powerfully anti-inflammatory. Certain bioflavonoids are believed to be anti-carcinogenic and the methoxylated bioflavonoid stops red blood cells clumping together, decreasing blood viscosity by as much as 6%.

All bioflavonoids are at their most powerful and active when the body is under stress; considering that many of them are useful for combating fungi, viruses and bacteria, this is a particularly desirable asset.

Nutritional Yeast

There are literally hundreds of different types of yeast that have various qualities. Many of the yeasts on the market today, however, are the by-products of manufacturing processes in the brewing industry (hence the name brewer's yeast) or designed for the baking industry. In the past some of these yeasts have been grown on rags and old newspapers; they are often used as food supplements. My feeling is that not only is their nutritional value suspect, but their quality is very poor and some are even toxic. Nature gives you a clue simply because they often taste and smell somewhat unpleasant and bitter. More importantly, they are still active, meaning they are alive, and can be damaging to those people who have yeast infections and/or overgrowth problems with *Candida albicans*.

Saccharomyces cerevasiae nutritional yeast, however, is grown solely for human consumption as a nutritional food supplement. It is cultivated on a base of pure beet and cane molasses and it absorbs this base in the same way as plants utilize minerals in the soil. Molasses is used because it provides the yeast with an abundant organic source of B vitamins and minerals. Once the yeast is harvested, it is thoroughly washed and dried and during the drying process it is heated just enough to stabilize it, thereby making it completely non-fermentable. This process not only makes the yeast incapable of any further fermentation in the digestive tract, but helps it to be easily digestible and assimilable. It is therefore particularly recommended for those with internal bacterial or fungal infections, including *Candida albicans*.

Garlic

Garlic, known botanically as *Allium sativum*, is one of nature's miracle foods. The ancient Egyptians, Greeks and Romans all used garlic copiously to increase strength and fight disease and illness. Hippocrates used garlic specifically to treat cancer. In the First World War the British government administered garlic in battlefield hospitals: it saved thousands of lives. It was used in numerous preparations to disinfect and heal battle wounds internally, and to treat typhoid fever and dysentery.

Today garlic is the leading over-the-counter drug in many European and Asian countries. It is an official drug in many countries and prescribed by medical doctors outside the US for many diseases, especially hypertension (high blood pressure), high cholesterol and cancer, and as a broad-spectrum antibiotic, antiviral agent and fungicide.

Garlic is famous for its healing power with heart disease. Countries where garlic consumption is high have a lower incidence of heart disease than average. Garlic lowers serum cholesterol and triglyceride levels and reduces the build-up of atherosclerotic plaque in our arteries. It does this partly by increasing the blood levels of high-density lipoproteins (HDLs). These lipoproteins clear the blood of excess cholesterol and fat. Garlic also lowers numbers of low-density lipoproteins (LDLs), which can contribute to arterial plaque. Medical researchers have also found substances in garlic that inhibit blood platelet aggregation (the sticking together of blood cells). Because of its powerful effect on blood pressure, the Japanese Food and Drug Administration has approved garlic and it is now an official drug listed in the Japanese Pharmacopoeia.

Garlic is an effective cancer therapy. One-third of all the medical research into garlic is cancer related. The National Cancer Institute has reported that cancer incidence worldwide is lowest in the countries where garlic consumption is highest. Garlic has been shown to help white blood cells combat cancer and increase the ability to destroy tumours. When the properties of garlic are present in the bloodstream, many aspects of our immunity are enhanced. Garlic has also been found to stimulate interferon production, enhance natural killer cells, stop tumour growth, and even reduce the associated pain of cancer. It has been found to reduce the incidence of colonic and rectal cancer and stomach cancer. In one medical university study garlic was shown to reduce stomach cancer ten times more effectively than in those who did not eat garlic. With over 80 different sulphur compounds, it is a free-radical scavenger. This is just another way that garlic protects from cancers, even those that are chemically induced.

Garlic juice diluted one part in 125,000 has been found to inhibit the growth of bacteria. Garlic destroys both gram positive and gram negative bacteria, making it a broad-spectrum antibiotic. Garlic used as an antibacterial agent in Russia is so revered it has been christened Russian penicillin. Unlike antibiotics, garlic is selective in its bacteria destruction, only killing bacteria that are harmful to the body. At the same time, it enhances our friendly bacteria and improves our intestinal flora and digestion.

Garlic destroys many types of bacteria including streptococcus, staphylococcus, typhoid, diphtheria, cholera, bacterial dysentery (traveller's diarrhoea), tuberculosis, tetanus, rheumatic bacteria and many others. Some say that the reason you don't catch colds when you eat garlic is because no one will come near you! Garlic is certainly a powerful antiviral agent. Many feel it's the cure for the common cold. It will destroy the different viruses that cause upper respiratory infections and influenza. Garlic has been shown to destroy on contact the viral infections of measles, mumps, mononucleosis, chickenpox, herpes simplex 1 and 2, herpes zoster, viral hepatitis, scarlet fever and rabies.

Garlic's antifungal ability is second to none. Laboratory tests have proved it to be more potent than any known antifungal agent, including Nystatin. Garlic will regulate the overgrowth of *Candida albicans*.

The Vitamin and Mineral Controversy

Nearly all vitamin and mineral supplements are currently not made from food. In fact, commercial vitamins and minerals are nearly always synthesized by the large pharmaceutical companies from exactly the same material that drugs are made from – coal tar derivatives, petrol products, animal by-products (including parts of their bodies and their faecal matter) and pulverized rocks, stones, shells and metals. The United States Pharmacopoeia simply says that if a product looks similar under a microscope or any other form of laboratory analysis it is the same product regardless of what it is made from. For example, salicylic acid is considered identical whether it comes from wintergreen leaves or from boiling coal in carbolic and sulphuric acid; glycerine may be made from fresh vegetable sources or boiled down animal carcasses, particularly the cartilage and hooves.

Synthesizing Synthetic Vitamins and Minerals

Vitamins and minerals naturally present in food are bound to food complexes with carbohydrates, proteins and lipids. The human body recognizes only this entire food complex as food. Nearly all supplements are synthetic combinations of isolated vitamins and minerals which are not bound to anything and may have an entirely different chemical structure from those found in food. They are also formulated so they can boast of 100% of the daily recommended allowance on their labels.

These synthetic formulae often ignore antagonistic and synergistic effects among vitamins and minerals, as far as both absorption and metabolic reactions are concerned. The chelating agent in wholefoods that assists absorption may be missing and synthetic calcium and iron are not well absorbed by humans.

Megadoses of vitamin and mineral supplements are largely excreted simply because the uptake mechanism in the intestines cannot cope with them, which is why B complex will turn urine yellow and make it smell strongly and iron will blacken the faeces. Megadosing is not simply a waste of money, it can also be dangerous. If the body relies on formulated supplements it is possible that it may get lazy or 'forget' how to extract the nutrients from food efficiently. In other words megadoses may actually block the body's normal and natural wisdom. Bear in mind too that the technology which bought us chemical chelators, transporters and time-release agents in an attempt to get round this problem, is in itself synthetic. Such concentrates may affect sensitive people.

It is better to get our nutrients from natural sources because our bodies are designed to absorb nutrients from food. It isn't just how much you take of a nutritional supplement that matters, it is how much you absorb. I have yet to find any synthetic vitamins and minerals which are compatible to the human digestive tract.

Most people are unaware that vitamin B_{12}, cyanocobalamin, is made from ground-up cow's livers or activated sewage sludge. These cow's livers are over-loaded already with steroids and antibiotics and the pesticides that cows ingest while eating. Vitamin A is made from fish livers and the toxic overload from these I have clearly outlined (see page 11). Vitamin D is made from radiated oil, vitamin C from acid blends which can irritate the lining of sensitive digestive tracts, and most minerals are simply made from pulverized and powdered shells and rocks. In today's environment where increasingly depressed immune systems are responsible for many serious illnesses I can think of hundreds of reasons why all of these materials would be a health risk rather than a benefit, hence my espousal of nature's Superfoods. (For suppliers see Resources Directory.)

6 AVOID EXCESSIVE PROTEIN

For too long now we have been held in thrall by the high-protein cult. World health statistics show that osteoporosis is most common in exactly those countries where dairy and flesh products are consumed in the largest quantities – the USA, Finland, Sweden and the UK. Two facts have been known for a long time.

- The Inuit diet, laden with fish, fish bones and meat, produces the osteoporosis champions of the world. Physically active vegans rarely suffer from osteoporosis.
- Vegans live longer than flesh eaters, who also suffer from higher rates of cancer of the breast, prostate, pancreas and colon.

HOW MUCH IS ENOUGH?

We grow faster during infancy on mother's breast milk than at any other time in our lives yet breast milk is only about 2–4% protein at birth; and it reduces to 1.2–1.6% within six months. Even as adults we need very little protein. Our bodies lose about 0.8 oz (22 g) daily, about 1½ lb (675 g) monthly. Various experts ranging from the *American Journal of Clinical Nutrition* to the World Health Organisation estimate optimum intake as between 2.5 and 8%. Interestingly, mother's milk falls pretty much halfway between these two – which just shows what a perfectly balanced food it is.

SOURCES OF PROTEIN

There is protein in practically everything we eat. Wheat, for example, is 17% protein, oatmeal 15%, cabbage 22%, pumpkin 15%, potato 11%. Arnold Schwarzenegger recommends 1 g protein for every 2 lb (900 g) of body weight and if you ate nothing but cabbage all day you would still be getting four times his suggested requirement (and probably very bored with a mono-diet!). So the idea that plant protein is somehow incomplete is a myth.

THE MYTH OF OSTEOPOROSIS

Milk is touted as a great natural source of calcium, and we are told to eat plenty of calcium to prevent osteoporosis. In fact, eating dairy products can increase the rate at which calcium is lost from the body and so hasten osteoporosis. As well as being high in calcium, dairy products are also high-protein foods. If you have too much protein in the diet – from milk products or other sources such as meat, fish or eggs – the body has to get rid of the excess. To do this, the kidneys must lose calcium as they cleanse the blood of excess waste, a process known as protein-induced hypercalciuria.

People in the United States and Scandinavian countries consume more dairy products than anyone else in the world, yet they have the highest rate of osteoporosis. This fact emphasizes the threat of excessive protein in the diet and suggests that dairy products offer no protection against osteoporosis, probably due to the high protein content of milk.

The body's ability to absorb and utilize calcium depends on the amount of phosphorus in the diet. The higher the calcium–phosphorus ratio, the less bone loss takes place and the stronger the skeleton, provided the intake of protein is not excessive. The foods which contain high calcium–phosphorus ratios are fruit and vegetables.

Cooked animal protein can cause serious health disorders. The metabolism of excessive protein in the diet leaves behind toxic residues of metabolic waste, causing self-poisoning, over-acidity and nutritional deficiencies, as well as an accumulation of uric acid and purines in the tissues. It encourages intestinal dysbiosis and contributes to the development of most of our chronic degenerative diseases, including arthritis, pyorrhoea, kidney damage, schizophrenia, osteoporosis, atherosclerosis, heart disease and cancer. A diet which is too high in protein accelerates the ageing process, so lowering life expectancy.

A study made by the US Army Medical Research and Nutrition Laboratory in Colorado demonstrated that the more meat eaten, the more deficient the body becomes in vitamins B_6 and B_3, as well as in magnesium, calcium and niacin. Mental illness and schizophrenia are often caused by niacin deficiency and have been treated successfully by high doses of niacin. Russian researchers have made great inroads with schizophrenia by placing sufferers on a low-protein diet. It seems that amyloid, a by-product of protein metabolism, is deposited in all the connective tissues, causing tissue and organ degeneration and so exacerbating the ageing process. This may explain why isolated tribes dotted around the world seem to have the highest average life expectancy. Ammonia, which is produced by eating meat, is carcinogenic. A high-protein diet tends to debilitate the pancreas and lower resistance to cancer, as well as contribute to the development of diabetes. So not only should all animal proteins be, at best, consumed in moderation, but excessive protein consumption, even from such sources as soya milk or vegetables, should be discouraged.

7 PURE WATER

It has become almost impossible to obtain uncontaminated natural water on our planet. Millions of people in Britain are currently drinking water contaminated with levels of toxic chemicals far in excess of international standards. So far, over 350 different manmade chemicals have been detected in British tap water.

Fluoride

About 10% of people in the UK and 50% in the USA are drinking fluoridated water, which has been associated with cancer, genetic disorders, brittle bones and mottled teeth. The problem is most of us over-consume fluoride from natural sources such as food and drink, as well as artifical ones like insecticides, anaesthetics and preservatives. The difficulty is that only half of all ingested fluoride can be excreted by the average healthy adult; children, diabetics and those with debilitated kidneys may retain as much as two-thirds of their ingested fluoride. This build-up in the body is associated with bone-related cancer, liver/bile cancer, oral lesions, abnormal cell changes and metaplasias (replacement of one tissue type with another). The link between fluoride and brittle bones has long been established but even very low levels of fluoride inhibit the ability of leucocytes (infection-fighting white blood cells) to migrate, which means fluoride depresses the immune system.

There are now water filters on the market that remove fluoride, if you live in a fluoridated area (see Resources Directory).

8 CLEANSING

Cleanse your system periodically with juice fasting. Systematic under-eating and periodic fasting are two of the most important health and longevity factors. Periodic juice fasting speeds up the process of elimination of toxic waste and accelerates and stimulates the building of new cells. It also normalizes all metabolic and nervous functions and increases cell oxygenation. Once the fast is broken, the digestion of food and utilization of nutrients is handled much more efficiently, and sluggishness and water retention are prevented, all of which has a far reaching effect on the body's ability to withstand stress and prevent disease.

Fasting: The Ultimate Detox

Fasting is undoubtedly the most powerful medicinal tool I use in my practice. Most therapeutic fasts last from three to seven days. The only liquid taken is mineral or purified water, fruit or vegetable juices and broths decocted from them.

Never subject a child to a fast, unless incontrovertible medical opinion prescribes it; get professional help if you think a fast may be a good idea for your child.

Fasting helps the body to heal itself by allowing the digestive tract to rest, by encouraging the mobilization of various detoxifying defence mechanisms and by stimulating consequent recuperation. The theory behind fasting is that the body is well equipped with mechanisms for eliminating nutritional waste, as well as the toxic effects of negative feelings (which may have more to do with the cause of illness than any other factor). Our digestive process uses up 30% of our entire body's energy so if the digestive system is allowed to rest completely that energy can be channelled to detoxification and healing. Fasting is a superb tool, both in emergencies and to accelerate the healing of long-term illnesses. If carried out on a regular basis, it can help to rebalance the body mentally, spiritually, physically and emotionally.

Fasting is also an invaluable preventative medicine. Not only does it help the body achieve physical peakness by periodically unburdening itself of accumulated waste, but it also prevents minor health problems from developing into major ones. Fasting slows down the ageing process, and helps the body to utilize nutrients far more effectively after the fast is broken.

If done on a regular basis, juice fasting can:

- lead to a longer more active life
- promote faster healing
- greatly reduce the risk of DNA damage
- enhance the ability to fight off potential carcinogens.

The uninitiated often think fasting will lead to stress and fatigue but in fact it does quite the opposite. I have found it the most potent, quick-acting antidote to lethargy and anxiety. I always emerge from a three-day or longer fast looking younger, with an even better skin, with my hair and nails in even better health, a few pounds lighter and with abundant energy.

I generally do not recommend fasting until the eliminative organs are working at their best levels and a patient has been following a diet high in alkaline foods including fruits, vegetables, nuts, grains and seeds, and excluding all animal produce (including eggs and dairy produce and fish), as well as avoiding alcohol, tea, coffee, anything white or refined and chemical drugs. If people leap into a fast without ensuring this is the case, they may experience discomfort and – unless the toxins are actively eliminated from the system – the fast is a complete waste of time and energy. A fast should be supported with plenty of hydrotherapy, enemas or colonics, bodywork of some sort and exercise.

How to Fast

A juicer is one of the first tools I insist anybody working with me purchases. I call the juicer 'nature's intravenous drip' because fasting with juices can alter the quality of the bloodstream more rapidly than any other method. Juices bought from health-food stores and supermarkets tend to be boiled and, therefore, leached of many of their nutrients, or they have preservatives added to them. Anything which is bottled and labelled organic is generally acceptable, although there are juices that are organic but contain whey. While fasting on these is better than not fasting at all, I would urge you to find a source of organic fruit and vegetables and juice them freshly as needed.

How Much is Enough?

When supervising patients through juice fasting, it is often difficult to get them to drink enough juice. You should aim to drink 1 fl oz (30 ml) of juice for every 1 lb (450 g) of your body weight every day. This means that you may well be drinking a gallon (4.5 litres) or more of liquid a day. The more liquid you ingest, the quicker you flush out all those accumulated toxins and the less possibility there is of retaining water, because mineral water or purified water and juices act as natural diuretics.

How to Juice

All juices should be served at room temperature and, if possible, pressed freshly as needed (to minimize oxidation). They should be well chewed before swallowing. You don't actually have to move your jaw to do this. Just swish them well around the mouth to ensure they are mixed with plenty of saliva before swallowing.

When juicing, remove the skins of oranges and grapefruits because they contain toxic substances that should not be consumed in large quantities. However leave on the white pithy part of the peel because it contains valuable bioflavonoids. Tropical fruits like kiwi and pawpaw should be peeled before pressing because they are grown in countries where carcinogenic sprays are still legal and used. The skins of all other fruits and vegetables, including lemons and limes, can be left as long as the fruit has not been waxed. All stones (peach, apricot, plum) should be removed before juicing, but seeds can be placed in the juicer with the fruit.

Those fruits and vegetables that contain little water, like bananas and avocados, cannot be juiced but can be used as an ingredient in a Fruit Smoothy.

FRUIT SMOOTHY

A Smoothy is fresh fruit juice liquidized with fresh and frozen fruit.

My favourite recipe is 8 fl oz (250 ml) of apple juice liquidized at high speed with one fresh banana and a cupful of frozen berries. Switch off the liquidizer when the whole mixture is creamy.

Before juicing wash all your produce well and remove any mouldy or bruised parts. Throw the excess pulp on to your compost heap if you have one. If for some reason you have to prepare juice in advance, store it in a thermos flask and fill it as near to the top as possible so there is no air left in the flask; add the juice of a lemon to inhibit oxidation. Try to make juice only from locally grown produce in its proper season. Juice will keep adequately in a thermos flask without fermenting for up to eight hours.

POTASSIUM BROTH

This is a very useful addition to a fast. Fill one quarter of a large pot with thickly cut potato peelings (¼ inch), then add equal amounts of carrot peelings and whole chopped beetroot, chopped onions and garlic, and celery and greens.

Add hot chili peppers to taste. Add enough water to cover the vegetables and simmer on very low heat for 1–2 hours. Strain and drink only the broth and put the vegetables on the compost. Make enough for two days (refrigerate leftover broth), then start a new broth.

Do not mix fruit and vegetable juices together as the enzymes in them are incompatible. The only exception to this rule is carrot and apple juice. Various types of juices will heal specific conditions and there are many helpful books about this.

Starting and Finishing a Fast

Ease into and out of a fast by eating fresh fruits and vegetables for one, two or three days before and afterward. Never shock the body by changing from a heavy diet to fasting or vice versa, unless you are fasting for first aid purposes.

If you have never fasted before, fast for between one and three days only. Fasting for longer than a week needs medical supervision from a professional experienced with the technique.

Breaking a fast is as important as the fast itself. You can undo most of the good of a fast by breaking it improperly or unwisely. Eat a home-made vegetable soup containing some well-cooked grains, or choose fresh fruit and, separately from the fresh fruit, a large raw salad lightly dressed with olive oil and lemon juice. Spend as long breaking a fast as the fast itself. So if the fast took three days, introduce solid foods gradually over a three-day period.

Do not be too rigid about how many days you are going to fast. I have started three-day fasts and gone on to ten days because I was feeling so wonderful, and I have also set out to do seven-day fasts and finished after 36 hours because I had had enough. But I find fasting easy – it involves requires less menu preparation (providing you haven't bought dirty carrots and have to spend all day at the sink scrubbing them) and eliminates the possibility of choice and hence temptation.

Fasting for more than a day actually lowers the metabolic rate and the spectacular amount of weight that is lost during the initial days of a fast is merely the result of the liver dumping glycogen and water levels adjusting in the body. A substantial percentage of the weight lost during a long fast is rapidly regained after normal eating has been resumed. This is reassuring for very thin people, not so good for the overweight. However, fasting, for those who want to lose weight, is a wonderful way to introduce you to taking control of your diet. It shores up willpower and shrinks the stomach so that smaller helpings will do; and digestion of any food eaten after a fast is greatly enhanced, and glandular chemistry and hormonal secretions are stimulated.

9 HEALTH-PROMOTING EATING HABITS

You should never eat when you are not hungry, you should not drink when you are not thirsty. Remember your requirements of food and drink are unique to you, so 'rules' don't apply.

Never eat when you are stressed. We require more than good nutrition to make us happy and healthy. Anger and resentment actually act like physical poisons in the body. Fear can compromise your immune system so much it will finally make you ill. So the dining room should never be a battleground. Eat slowly and masticate thoroughly. Good chewing increases the assimilation of nutrients and makes you feel satisfied with smaller amounts of food. Saliva well mixed with food contains enzymes which are essential for proper digestion.

Do not eat cooked foods late at night, this stresses the body at a time when it wants to rest and sleep.

It is far better to eat four, five or even six small meals a day than two or three large ones. This stabilizes your blood sugar levels. It is also interesting to note that 2,000 calories eaten in two meals may result in new fat accumulation, while 2,000 calories eaten in six small meals with two- or three-hour intervals in between will not only fail to add weight but may actually help you to burn up the food more efficiently and so lose weight.

Do not mix too many foods at the same meal. There is much cumulative evidence to the effect that the fewer foods you mix at any one meal the better your digestion and assimilation will be. In his ground-breaking book *The Work of the Digestive Glands* (1902) Ivan Pavlov proved that every kind of food provides a specific definite type of gastric and intestinal secretion. Because the presence of three concentrated foods (protein, carbohydrate and fruit, for example) calls for antagonistic chemical processes at the same time, it is a physical and a chemical impossibility for the digestive glands to function properly because they are governed by definite laws. So if you want to assimilate your food and make full use of it, it needs to be ingested in specific and optimum combinations.

If we don't do this, the partially digested food can produce harmful toxins which place all sorts of strains on a body trying to offload the poison. In addition, the one process that uses the most energy in our body is digestion. It takes up more energy than running, swimming or cycling. So if we treat our digestive processes kindly, our organs will not be prematurely exhausted.

Starchy foods (like rice, barley, wheat and potatoes) need an alkaline environment for digestion. Proteins (nuts, soya beans) need an acid solution for digestion. If you mix a starchy food and a protein together (dates and nuts, eggs and chips, beans on toast) both acid and alkaline digestive solutions are simultaneously produced. They neutralize each other and digestion grinds to a halt or, at best, is impaired. The starches ferment, causing a souring of the stomach and gas and if you keep this up you may develop a stomach ulcer.

If you wake up exhausted, even after seven or eight hours of solid sleep every night, you may well be hypoglycaemic (see page 177), but you may simply feel that way because your long-suffering digestion has been doing the graveyard shift trying to digest the incompatible mess sloshing around inside you. This can go on for 14 hours; properly combined foods digest in only three or four hours.

- Try to eat only one concentrated food in a meal, that is, any food that is not water rich. Water-rich foods embrace all fruit and vegetables except squashes, pumpkin, potatoes and legumes, which count as concentrated foods because they are more dense and solid.
- Do not eat protein and starch mixed together.
- Do not mix fruit and starch. In fact all fruit should be eaten in isolation and on an empty stomach. This is because it is so high in water and, as such, incredibly cleansing and leaves behind no toxic residue. It is easy to digest. It doesn't in fact digest in the stomach, but is predigested and sweeps through the stomach in 20 minutes, releasing its supercharged nutrients into the small intestine and bloodstream. Fruit juice acts even more rapidly as an energy boost.
- Do not mix raw fruits and vegetables in the same meal because their enzyme combinations are incompatible for digestion. The exceptions are carrot and apple which combine well together. Avocado (strictly a fruit) can be counted as a vegetable.

All this applies to fresh fruit and freshly squeezed juices. Baked, canned, stewed or dried fruit does not have the same nutritional value, nor does cooked or prepacked juice. Allow 20 to 30 minutes to pass before putting anything else into your stomach and leave three to four hours to elapse if you have previously eaten anything other than fresh fruit.

Under-eat systematically because overeating is the main cause of disease and premature ageing. Overeating is particularly dangerous for older people, who are less active and whose metabolism has slowed.

10 AVOID THE HEALTH DESTROYERS

Some of these are evident from what I have said previously, but others are so obvious they need no explanation.

- All tobacco and passive smoking.
- Coffee, tea, chocolate, cola drinks and refined drinks – soft drinks, squashes, cordials and anything fizzy.
- Excessive use of salt.
- Excessive consumption of alcohol.
- Too many spices including mustard, black and white pepper and distilled vinegar. (A little cider vinegar or lemon juice is acceptable.)
- Anything refined, especially white flour and anything made with it.
- All processed, refined, canned or manufactured foods.
- All rancid foods: baked goods may be an obvious source but some health foods such as wheatgerm, seeds and vegetable oils need to be refrigerated once bought.
- All chemical drugs except on a doctor's advice and in an emergency.
- All household and environmental toxic chemicals including dry-cleaned clothes (hang in the fresh air first) as well as more obvious garden sprays and household cleaners.

- Lack of sufficient exercise and relaxation. Not only does exercise keep the eliminative organs working effectively, but it also tones the muscles, improves digestion and general metabolism, activates better circulation and encourages optimum function of all organs and glands, and increases and improves tissue oxygenation. The bedrock of disease and premature ageing is lack of oxygen in the cells so vigorous daily exercise keeps all the cells and tissues well oxygenated and at peak efficiency.

In my opinion, all disease springs from stress and a troubled and unresolved mind. Fear, anxiety, worry, tension, depression, hate, jealousy, unhappiness, lack of love, isolation and loneliness can cause every disease known; by contrast, a contented spirit, some kind of spiritual philosophy, lots of giving and receiving of love, as well as the absence of envy and jealousy and an optimistic outlook are all powerfully health promoting.

SUGGESTIONS FOR A HEALTHY DAILY DIET

On rising, drink a glass of pure filtered water, slightly warmed if desired, with freshly squeezed lime, lemon or grapefruit juice in it, or a large mug of herbal tea or a glass of freshly squeezed fruit juice from any whole fruits in season. The juice should be diluted half and half with pure water. (Do not use canned or frozen juices.) Squeeze it freshly in your juicer just before drinking.

Take at least 40 minutes' brisk aerobic exercise combined with deep breathing and any stretching you can manage to fit in. If you live on a farm or own a garden, this is the ideal time to get in an hour's hard physical work to get your metabolism going. On your return from your exercise, skin brush vigorously (see page 87) and follow this with the seven times hot/cold shower routine (see page 50). You are now ready for breakfast.

BREAKFAST

Fresh fruits of any sort organically grown in your own locality and environment, and in season. If you are very hungry add to this, after a 20-minute wait, sprouted seeds or a bowl of pre-soaked, low-heated (and therefore uncooked) rolled oats or pot millet with pre-soaked dried fruit and oat or rice milk added. Digest this for two to three hours before having as much freshly squeezed fruit juice and herbal tea to drink until midday as you desire.

Alternatively, have a Fruit Smoothy or banana milk.

FRUIT SMOOTHY

10 oz (285 g) frozen fruit
1 fresh banana, peeled, or any other soft fruit in season
1 cup of frozen seasonal or fresh berries
2 tbsp Superfood (optional)
Liquidize until smooth and creamy.

BANANA MILK

> *3 sliced ripe bananas*
> *2 cups ice-cold water*
> *1½ tbsp tahini*
> *1 tbsp maple syrup, barley malt or other sweetener (optional)*
> *½ tsp natural vanilla*
> *Liquidize until smooth and creamy.*

LUNCH

- A large bowl of freshly prepared fruit salad (if not eaten for breakfast)
- Freshly prepared vegetable soup or any other cooked vegetable dish with one or two slices of wholegrain bread
- Some rice cakes with vegetable pâté
- A large salad with baked potatoes and an interesting vegetable filling
- Pasta (try corn or rice pasta not wheat pasta) with an interesting sauce and a large side salad

One of my favourite salad dressings, which is both tasty and nutritious, is two-thirds organic cold-pressed olive oil, one-third cider vinegar or freshly squeezed lemon juice, a generous teaspoon of grainy mustard, a teaspoon of maple syrup (preferably organic) or runny honey (preferably organic), two cloves of garlic and a heaped tablespoon of Engevita yeast liquidized together. Alternatively, omit the garlic and add freshly chopped herbs to your taste. This keeps very well in a screw-top jar in the fridge.

MID-AFTERNOON

A glass of fresh fruit or vegetable juice or a cup of herbal tea or fresh fruit, or a tub of soya yogurt with fresh fruit chopped into it.

DINNER

Try to keep this lighter than lunch and include, if you haven't had it for lunch, a large bowl of salad with sprouted seeds. (Carrots, shredded beetroot and onions should be staples in every salad.) Or a bowl of homemade soup with handfuls of sprouted seeds sprinkled into it and some oat or rice cakes to go with it. Try not to eat cooked food later than 7–8 p.m. and, if hungry beyond this time, take fruit or vegetable juice or fresh fruit.

BEDTIME

For a bedtime snack you can have a glass of freshly made nut milk or rice or oat milk with maple syrup and honey if desired or hot 'chocolate' made with organic soya milk and carob powder.

POINTS TO REMEMBER

- Whatever changes you make, bear in mind that the bulk of your diet should consist of seeds, nuts and grains and fresh vegetables and fruits, especially organically grown; up to 80% of them, ideally, should be eaten raw. Eat the widest variety of available foods possible, but not in the same meal.
- Lunch and dinner menus are interchangeable, but keep dinner lighter.
- Remember to eat at least one large vegetable meal a day.
- Separate your protein and carbohydrate in any one meal.
- Do not drink liquids with a meal unless they are freshly squeezed vegetable juices or organic bottled vegetable juices or herbal teas (which could be medicinal).
- Drink between meals or 15 minutes before meals and try and ensure that you have at least six glasses of pure water a day. The brain is 85% water so if you are starting to feel headachy or tired it is a very good idea to rehydrate yourself on pure, non-carbonated, water. Carbonated water is more difficult to assimilate, as the gas pumped into it is precisely the same as the waste gas you are breathing out. Take carbonated water as fun liquidation; the serious option is plain filtered water.

ELIMINATE	SUBSTITUTE
Salt	Flavourful kitchen herbs, spices, seaweeds, soya sauce, miso, sesame salt. Sesame salt is easy to make and stretches the saltiness of the salt. The ratio is eight parts sesame meal to one part salt. Simply stir sesame meal constantly in a heavy bottomed frying pan until thoroughly heated through and toasted. Decant. Now, heat up the salt and return the toasted sesame, stirring the mixture until well amalgamated. Decant again. Cool and store in a cupboard container.
Tea, coffee, alcohol	Herbal teas, dandelion coffee (avoid the ones with lactose added), grain coffees, potassium broth, warmed juices, miso, fresh juices. Both tea and coffee are high in tannin which neutralizes iron, so both need to be eliminated when taking herbal supplements.
Sugar	Honey, maple syrup, dried fruits, date syrup, carob, fruit juices and sweet root vegetables.
Meat, fish, chicken, eggs	Tofu, nuts, seeds, spirulina, chlorella, Engevita yeast, high-protein substitutes made of soya.

ELIMINATE	SUBSTITUTE
Dairy products	Soya products, nut milks, rice and oat milks. Note that all dairy products can be substituted by soya, including ice-cream, cheese, yogurt, milk, custard and cream.
Flour, pasta	Because wheat flour is mucus-forming, use chickpea, millet, spelt, quinoa, soya or rice flour. Try corn or rice pasta, not wheat pasta. If using wheat flour, opt for wholegrain fresh organic flour products without chemical additives and preservatives.
Carbonated fizzy drinks, fruit squashes, sugar-sweetened drinks, concentrated juices	Filtered water with a dash of citrus to cheer up the flavour, if desired, herbal teas, fresh fruits and vegetable juices, potassium broth and miso.

CRAVINGS

Unless you are in a life-or-death situation it is important to enjoy the foods you love or crave. If you hold yourself under a very tight rein for too long, it is inevitable that you will fall over the edge into a binge or reverse entirely into negative-eating patterns. In my many years in practice I have heard people lamenting the fact that they indulge in chocolate, cream, coffee, ice cream, alcohol, bread or toast and jam in excess when they are feeling low. Ultimately the foods they crave actually increase the imbalance of the liver which is lulled by chewing on soft sweet carbohydrates or dairy products. The Superfoods, particularly spirulina and chlorella, will help to reduce craving. In addition, meditation, acupuncture, shiatsu and the practice of some of the Chinese martial arts may be helpful. Chewing helps too, because the jaw gets tight with emotions or distress. Alleviate this by chewing on sunflower seeds. They are very high in B vitamins and various minerals and reasonably low in calories. As the body starts to rebalance itself, cravings diminish.

I have one final piece of advice on diet reform. **Don't do it all at once**. Alter one aspect of your diet at a time, unless you are in a life-or-death situation and have no time to waste. Choose to give up, say, coffee to start with, and expect to feel exhausted initially as you come off its adrenal-stimulating qualities. Use herbal help to cleanse and support the body while you do so.

Once you have transferred your allegiance to an imaginative, balanced, wholefood, predominantly raw diet, you will notice that your tastebuds get sharper and fussier and there will come a time when you actually feel nauseated rather than guilty when you eat foods that don't suit you. Alternatively, you will get headaches, aches and pains, a rash, diarrhoea, bloodshot eyes or halitosis and you will decide that the food is simply not worth it. Don't become a fanatic but don't let other people's opinions bother or sway you. Stay with your helpful friends as far as diet reform is concerned. Avoid your unhelpful ones until the pattern of your life is comfortable with your chosen way of eating.

Once you have cut out the junk food from your diet and cleared the rubbish from your system, there will come a time when your body will be intelligent enough to tell you instinctively what it needs. I have worked with people who have vomited even a cup of herbal tea at the beginning of any dietary reform. This is because the body is so toxic, and the digestion so battered, that it cannot deal even with the simplest element of pure nutrition. In such instances I get a patient to start with a few teaspoons of the tea and graduate from there. Accurate instincts about diet only begin once you have cleaned out the body. At first you will find that instinct appears in fits and starts because the new way of eating is rather like learning to ride a bicycle. You tend to wobble about a lot and fall off several times, but if you are persistent and keep remounting you eventually get the hang of it. In the end the speed, once you have mastered it, is wonderfully exhilarating!

DIET, BABIES AND CHILDREN

I have witnessed untold battles at the dinner table; they are painful. The vital thing to remember is that your baby (and child) will do not what you tell him or her to do, but copy what they see you doing. The way to introduce your child to solid foods is to eat high-quality, whole natural foods yourself and, right from the start, keep nothing in the house which you wouldn't want your child to eat. Also trust your child's instincts. I have never, in my years of clinical practice (and I have treated thousands of babies and children), seen a child starve to death! There are many studies carried out with babies and small children which show that provided they are offered only good-quality foods, they are perfectly capable of choosing an excellent diet by themselves. Such a diet may look erratic to an adult, nut butter and bread one day and bananas the next, but a child's inner wisdom in choosing is superb.

I have witnessed many embarrassing situations over children's eating. An anxious parent tries to force a child to eat and naturally the child rebels. So the parent caves in and begins to offer titbits of junk food to tempt the child into eating. Quickly the child learns that the one way in which he or she can express independence and exercise some power over anxious parents is to rebel. This is precisely how a fussy eater is created. He or she then holds the whole family to ransom with erratic behaviour, while the nervous parents worry that the child is going to starve to death. Hang in there and offer a variety of high-quality food. Have bowls of fruit available between meals and eventually your child will come around. Fruit consumption varies enormously and seems to be tied into growth spurts.

Never use food as a bribe, reward or compensation for good behaviour. It should be for nourishment and pleasure.

Before the first birthday introduce as many foods as possible raw and liquidized. After that, introduce steamed and puréed vegetables, boiled and mashed potatoes, pre-soaked low-heated grains which are then liquidized, and pulses. Young children are particularly fond of sprouted seeds after their teeth have come through, because they are satisfying to chew. Introduce grains one at a time to check for allergic reactions. Buckwheat, millet and rice are usually fine; wheat sometimes causes problems. Salads and vegetables are often unpopular among young children, so it is a good idea to liquidize raw vegetables. One of my favourite recipes is for the Spanish tomato soup, gazpacho, which is easy to made. I usually pour mine over a base of wholewheat liquidized breadcrumbs soaked in a little lemon juice and olive oil. I have never had a young child reject this adult version of a liquidized salad!

Snacks between meals can be healthy. Try halva made with grape juice instead of sugar (available from health-food shops), home-made ice cream (freeze a banana, then liquidize it at high speed), fruit-juice ice-lollies, corn pops in olive oil, dried unsulphured fruit and home-made biscuits and cake.

When making biscuits and cakes at home try to use maple syrup, blackstrap unsulphured molasses or honey. Avoid sugar. Remember that some prepacked cereals are almost 50% sugar, as are carbonated drinks. Most children don't like tea or coffee, but they do like chocolate, which interferes with their calcium metabolism and damages the liver. It is also high in copper, which can contribute to the development of diabetes. Carob is a better substitute. Most young children don't like strong spices, salt, black pepper or mustard, so don't try to introduce them.

Remember that food prepared and served with love in a happy, peaceful environment is more nutritious than even the best-quality food served in a gritted-teeth atmosphere. And remember that it is not what you eat but what you assimilate that counts. Assimilation will be enhanced if the whole family enjoys eating together (or separately) in a loving and positive atmosphere.

CHAPTER 2

HERBAL PHARMACY

____

TYPES OF PREPARATION

Because a lot of disease begins with a malfunctioning digestive system it is important to know how to administer herbs to yourself or others in alternative ways. In the West, we tend to think that we must eat something medicinal to make ourselves well, but it is pointless giving herbs to somebody whose digestive tract is working so poorly that they are unable to swallow them. Happily there are a number of ways of correcting the balance of the body without orally ingesting any herbs.

- Smelling herbs by inhaling the vapour of essential oils put into boiling water or breathing in the fumes from burning oils (this was used in ancient times for healing the respiratory tract, with coltsfoot and mullein particularly popular, although it is an uncomfortable process and I wouldn't particularly recommend it). Essential oils can also be rubbed into pulse points in the skin, and then smelled. A carrier base of beeswax, lanolin or nut oil works best. The oil can also be rubbed directly inside the nose, although because nasal membranes are very sensitive it is much more comfortable to stir it into some sort of salve, so diluting its action. In India various mental diseases are treated with essential oils in this way, apparently very successfully.
- Introducing liquid into the anus, vagina, ears or nose, or inserting tampons soaked in herbal preparation, or a pessary made of herbs in a carrier base such as coconut oil.
- Applying herbs on to the skin by administering poultices or fomentations, rubbing in creams, ointments or oils, often accompanied by special massage movements, or even using the herbs infused or decocted in water (although other carrier bases, such as cider vinegar or milk, are employed from time to time). Using herbs to bathe only certain parts of the body, as when using an eye bath or soaking the feet or hands only. Warming the body by steaming in the evaporation from herbs put into boiling water. It is generally sensible to try to apply a remedy to the affected face area: that is the mouth, ears, nose or eyes.
- Gargling with herbs and then spitting them out.
- Massaging herbs into the gums, usually in powdered or tincture form, and leaving them there.

EXTERNAL BODY TREATMENTS

These can be administered in water, alcohol, oil and vinegar, although occasionally other substances, such as milk, are used.

WATER-BASED PREPARATIONS

Taken internally, such preparations are known as teas, but externally are called baths, poultices or fomentations. Bear in mind while this may be the simplest way to prepare herbs, the liquid will only contain the water-soluble principles of the plant. If used conscientiously over a period of time, the water-based preparation can be extremely effective and works especially well in young children. It often has a discernible effect within a few minutes, which is why hand and foot baths are only conducted over a five to eight minute period.

Fresh herbs should be crushed to break down the cellulose of the plant, which releases the active principles. Use a stainless steel knife, your fingers or a pestle and mortar to do this. Dried herbs should be chopped or pounded in a pestle and mortar. Alternatively, put the herbs in a sealed plastic bag and pound with a rolling pin. Remember that water-based herbal preparations decompose rapidly so they need to be made fresh each day. The exception to this is a decoction of the herbs boiled for 10 to 20 minutes before being strained out of the liquid. Such prolonged boiling is usually only used for roots, barks and berries and helps to preserve the herbal mixture for three to four days. Delicate parts of the herb, like the flowers, leaves and stamens, need to be steeped in water for 20 minutes. Use 1 oz (30 g) of the herb (remember that fresh herbs take up three or four times the room that dried ones do) and pour over them 1 pt (575 ml) freshly boiled filtered water which has first been allowed to stand for 30 seconds. If you use water that is actually boiling, it will be too harsh and destroy the potency of the herbs. Then stir the preparation thoroughly with anything that is not aluminium. Cover the container closely and leave to steep for 15 minutes, then strain through muslin, nylon, a stainless steel or silver tea-strainer or, for a large quantity of herbs, a fine sieve.

Seeds, roots, bark or very tough leaves like bay leaves need vigorous processing to make them surrender their medicinal properties. Their cell walls are so strong that more heat is needed than for flowers, leaves and stamens to ensure that the active constituents are transferred into the water.

Put 1 oz (30 g) of the herbs in the bottom of a glass, enamel or stainless steel saucepan, add 1 pt (575 ml) filtered water and cover with a tight-fitting lid. Bring to the boil and simmer very gently until the water is reduced by half; this generally takes about 15 minutes. Strain and use as required.

Should you need to use both the tough parts of the herb and the flowers in one mixture, it is better to make an infusion and decoction separately and then combine them. An infusion is the term used for preparing easily damaged herbs and a decoction used for the more rigorous process of boiling up tough herbs. All seeds, roots and bark need to be well crushed using a pestle and mortar or coffee grinder; burdock root and cinnamon only need steeping in freshly boiled, not boiling, water; valerian root should be steeped in cold water for 24 hours to ensure that the valerianic acid and essential oils are not lost. Decoctions will stay fresh for three to four days while infusions tend to only last for a day and a half at most.

Store what you do not need immediately in the refrigerator in a glass jar covered with muslin or linen to allow the water-based preparation to breathe (do not use plastic). Fine bubbles popping up to the surface are a sign that the preparation has begun to ferment, so throw it away – your garden will be grateful for it! However, if you make only 1 pt (575 ml) at a time you will generally find you finish the mixture within a day or so, so this should not be a problem.

ALCOHOL-BASED PREPARATIONS

The advantages of these are, first, that alcohol is a better solvent than water on certain types of plant constituents and, second, that they can be kept indefinitely if properly stored. An alcohol-based preparation is known as a tincture.

Use good-quality brandy, gin or vodka. Never use alcohol in the form of surgical spirit or methanol as these are poisonous when drunk. All alcohol needs to be at least 30% proof. In general you will find that the final amount of alcohol is only one-third of the original amount by volume as any herbs used, once strained out, absorb much of it. (My teacher, Richard Schulze, in the United States has started to make what he calls 'industrial strength' tinctures and does so by filling the entire jar with herbs and then covering it with alcohol. He uses only organically grown or wild-crafted herbs for all of his tinctures, and made in this way, their efficacy is extraordinary.) The conventional way to make a tincture is to use one-third of powdered or very finely chopped herbs to two-thirds alcohol by volume. Some herbalists use one-third alcohol and two-thirds water but I find this less effective. Combine 5 oz (140 g) powdered or very finely chopped herbs with 1 pt (575 ml) alcohol. Keep the container somewhere warm, an airing cupboard is ideal. Shake vigorously at least once daily (twice if you have the time) and strain through muslin after 14 days.

Tinctures should be started with a new moon and strained with a full moon 14 days later. The power of the waxing moon helps extract the medicinal properties. In her *Moon and Plant* (Society for Cancer Research, Arlesheim, 1975), Agnes Fyfe discusses the moon's nodal cycle in relation to both the earth and the plants on it. Over her lifetime she conducted 70,000 consecutive single tests on plant sap which proved irrefutably that the moon has a chartable influence on the way the sap rises and falls in plants. She was aware that medicinal plants were gathered in the past at particular times according to some faculty and knowledge now lost. Her experiments prove that such practices were not simply arcane but vital if herbs were to be used at their most effective. You can buy diaries which chart the course of the moon in your local stationery shop.

If there are still bits floating around in the tincture once you have strained it through muslin, strain it a second time through coffee filter paper (preferably unbleached) and cap the resulting mixture tightly. For external use tinctures can be rubbed on to the skin directly or applied on poultices previously dampened with water. Applying tincture of plantain to insect stings or bites and rubbing myrrh tincture into a gum boil, for example, are extremely effective.

EXTERNAL TREATMENTS

There are several ways in which herbal preparations are applied.

POULTICES

These may seem rather old fashioned but they are, in fact, a very useful form of treatment for external wounds or grazes, for ulcers and for drawing out boils. Additionally, they supply nutrients to the skin through lymphatic and blood circulatory systems to the tissues and organs beneath. Poultices are also a good way of softening and dispersing material that has become hardened, such as breast lumps. They are also very effective on limbs being treated for varicosity, thread veins, eczema, psoriasis and ulcerous conditions. You need:

- Herbs: fresh herbs need to be liquidized in a little water at high speed, while dried ones should be macerated (soaked) in a little hot water. Powdered ones can stay as they are.
- Use slippery elm powder, cornflower or arrowroot as a carrier base.
- Cider vinegar, preferably organic.
- A fine white cloth. Depending on the size of the area to be treated, a large handkerchief is often ideal, but for a large area gauze is also suitable and is available from chemists everywhere.
- Two large plates and a large saucepan of boiling water.
- Plastic sheeting such as a piece of bin bag or any large clean piece of plastic or clingfilm. You will also need to have on standby a supply of stretchy cotton bandages (the amount depends on the area to be treated: applying a poultice to the whole of the abdomen, for example, is going to take a lot more bandage than a poultice applied to your wrist) and safety pins.

Estimate how much of the herb you will need to treat to a depth of ¼ in (6 mm). Mix the herb with an equal quantity of your chosen carrier base and add enough cider vinegar, a little at a time, to form a thick paste. Mix in a china or glass basin with a stainless steel or wooden spoon. Spread out the piece of cotton on a plate over a saucepan of boiling water. Scrape the mixture on to one half of the cotton only, keeping it from the edge so that it does not squelch out when you use it. Fold the other half of the cotton over the top and press the edges together. Cover the whole poultice with the other plate and allow it to become hot. Remove it and apply as hot as is bearable to the affected area (do not burn yourself). Cover the poultice with plastic and secure it with bandages and then safety pins, or if the area is very large, a thin towel. Leave it on all night. If the poultice is to be applied somewhere on the trunk, wear a tight-fitting cotton teeshirt to hold it firmly in place.

Next morning peel your poultice off and wrap it up again using the plate method. While waiting for it to warm, cleanse the area by bathing it with half and half diluted cider vinegar and hot water. Re-apply the poultice but this time use the other side against the skin. Repeat again in the evening using a completely fresh poultice and re-using the other side again in the morning until the area is healed. The poultice needs to be refreshed and the contents inside the old poultice thrown away every 24 hours. The cloth used for the poultice can simply be scraped free of its contents, rinsed, boiled and dried for repeat use.

Mini-poultices are useful for treating outdoor emergencies such as bites and stings. Chew the relevant herb and mix it with plenty of saliva until it is soft and mushy. Spread this liquid herbal paste directly on to the swelling and, if you have it to hand, cap it with a piece of plastic or cotton to hold it in place until you can get indoors to do a proper job. Equal parts of cayenne pepper and plantain work well to draw out splinters, for example.

COMPRESSES

These are like dilute poultices designed to be used over very large areas. They assist the circulation of the lymph or blood to a specific area, so relieving swellings like varicose veins, goitres and muscular aches. Cold compresses ease head congestion, insomnia, fever, indigestion, sprains, bruises and sore throats. Many of my patients grumble about going to bed accompanied by the unromantic rustle of plastic bin bags (the plastic is necessary to hold in moisture from the compress), but having applied them faithfully they finish up agreeing that they are extremely effective. Compresses have the added advantage of often giving almost instant pain relief. As well as being made from fresh, dried or powdered herbs, they can be made from warmed oils, plant juices or tinctures diluted in water. Plant juices can be extracted from mucilaginous plants such as comfrey or aloe vera, by putting them through a juicer.

Hot Compresses

Make a double-strength herbal decoction by using 2 oz (50 g) herbs to 1 pt (575 ml) water and strain, mashing the herbs well down in the sieve to extract all the goodness from them. (Powdered herbs are particularly effective for this.) Reheat the liquid and dip into it white, pure cotton cloths (bits of old sheet will do nicely), wringing them out lightly but firmly. Wrap around the parts to be treated and secure with bandages and clingfilm or a piece of some other plastic. This will keep the moist heat of the compress intact and protect the bed sheets from seeping dampness. You may also need to protect the bed with a towel to prevent staining, especially if you are leaving the compress on all night.

If the compress needs to be reused, the simplest way is to turn a slow cooker or saucepan on high and drop in the damp compress, leaving the lid off. The compress will heat up very quickly and if you need to alternate compresses one can be kept hot and within reach in this way while the other is being used. If applying a compress for more than an hour it may be necessary to refresh it with enough herbal decoction or infusion to re-dampen it.

If you are treating a whole arm or a leg with the compress, soak either cotton tights or a long cotton glove in the herbal mixture. This cuts down on bandages which, if they have to be wrapped all the way up the arm, puttee style, are often awkward to remove. Silk stockings, although difficult to find, are a good alternative to cotton tights, although any natural fibre will do.

If you need to apply a compress to your trunk, use a close-fitting white cotton teeshirt. You will need to sustain the heat over the area concerned for as long as you can with hot water bottles. Do not use an electrical heating pad.

Cold Compresses

These are made in exactly the same way as hot ones, but allow the liquid to go cold before dipping the cloths in. A cold compress is generally applied for between 5 and 15 minutes and encourages the blood to move quickly to the surface in cases of high temperature, sprains and bruises. For fever it is necessary to change the compress every 5 to 10 minutes as it heats up. A cold compress left on for 20 to 30 minutes will relieve indigestion and insomnia and may be repeated if necessary once every two hours. A cold compress left on all night will relieve a sore throat and bring down the swelling, and is also particularly effective for swollen joints. Cold compresses can also be used in conjunction with applications of hot water. For example, a cold compress applied to the back of the neck at the same time as you take a hot foot bath relieves headaches and congestion, particularly sinus congestion, very quickly. Hot and cold compresses, three minutes of the hot and two minutes of the cold, are often used alternatively for the first 48 hours of an injury until healing is complete and are especially effective for sprained ankles.

BATHS

Therapeutic baths should last for only 2 to 10 minutes. They are not at all like the long luxurious baths you treat yourself to at home. Very hot immersion baths, if taken daily, encourage debility, mental lethargy, physical weakness, poor circulation and even depression.

The best way to take a hot bath is to enjoy a deep, hot one, interspersing it with showers of ice-cold water. If you do not have a shower as part of your bath, use one of those rubber ones you can purchase from a chemist and attach it directly to the tap. If you have a mixer tap and such an apparatus won't fit, have a couple of large plastic buckets of cold water on standby.

The only instance in which prolonged hot baths may be beneficial in medical terms is if they are taken when menstruation is late, for dysmenorrhoea (painful menstruation) as an antispasmodic, or as a pyretic for the treatment of fevers.

Herbal Baths

Add 1 gallon (4.5 litres) of strained herbal decoction or infusion to a half-filled bath. Immerse as much as possible of the body under the water for 15 to 20 minutes, protecting the head on a folded towel or bath pillow to make a comfortable resting place.

Clean the skin before you take the bath by vigorous skin brushing (see page 87) and wash any really dirty bits with a natural soap or flannel. Never use soap after any sweating therapy as it prevents the cholesterol coming out through the pores. Depending on the herbs used, herbal baths are extremely effective for insomnia, for quickly reducing acute pain such as that induced by strained or pulled muscles or cramping, and for the unbearable itch of eczema, poison oak or nettle rash.

Epsom Salt Baths

This treatment is not to be used for people suffering from high blood pressure or heart conditions but it is an excellent way of dispersing acidity from the system, soaking up aches and pains, getting the skin to work properly, inducing a short sweat for therapeutic purposes and cleansing the system of fungus. It is also a wonderfully effective bath to be taken at the onset of a cold and is particularly beneficial for any kind of deep purification and healing. I have used them often over the years in my own practice for people who are particularly toxic, especially those suffering from heavy metal poisoning. Epsom salt baths need to be taken on alternate days for six days, resting on the seventh day and on this day detoxifying the body with a fast on fruit or fruit juices.

Buy more than 1 lb (450g) of Epsom salts and mix it with enough almond oil to give it the texture of wet sea sand. Carry this into the bathroom in a large basin and rest it on the side of the bath. Now plug the bath while it is empty and stand in it massaging yourself all over with this mixture, using small circular movements working upward toward the heart. This exfoliates dead skin. Let the salts and oil fall into the empty bath and step out, then fill the bath as deeply as possible with hot water, adding an additional generously heaped cup of Epsom salts and one of cider vinegar (don't worry about the dead skin cells, they are invisible to the naked eye and will, anyway, disappear down the plug hole when you drain the bath away). Stir with your hands to dissolve the salts thoroughly and soak yourself in the bath for 30 minutes, adding more hot water as it cools. While you do so, sip as many cups of any diuretic herbal tea as you can (ginger mixed with a little maple syrup and lemon is my favourite, but peppermint and elderflower are also particularly pleasant tasting). Elimination through the skin is vital. Normally the skin does only one-twentieth of the work of the kidneys but by speeding it up with herbs and hydrotherapy it can take on one-tenth of their work, so relieving the kidneys of any added burden.

Have some ice cubes on standby in a bowl and a couple of flannels to apply to the face, neck and forehead if you feel dizzy, faint or sick. While the water is draining out of the bath, run a cold shower over your face and body to encourage it to cool down thoroughly. Alternatively, fill up plastic buckets with cold water and pour it over your body. Go to bed warmly dressed in natural fabric and pack yourself round with hot water bottles to encourage free perspiration. Some of my patients sweat so profusely that they need to get up in the middle of the night to change into fresh nightwear, which is all to the good. Don't wear any kind of body lotion or oil after this treatment. It will stop the skin breathing freely. If you are using a deodorant make sure that it is a natural one. Take a hot shower followed by a cold one the next morning or (preferably) take seven hot/cold showers finishing up with a cold one (see page 50).

Salt Glow

This is an effective way of dislodging superficial catarrh in the tissues and I recommend patients of mine who suffer from chronic catarrh which nothing seems to move to carry it out three to four times a week. I have found it extremely successful.

Stand naked in an empty shower tray and shower the skin all over with warm water. Mix 1 lb (450g) fine salt with enough water to turn it into a soft slurry and pick up palmfuls of this at a time massaging vigorously into the skin with brisk circular movements. Start with the soles of the feet, moving upward toward the heart. Areas above the heart should be massaged downward toward the heart. Do not massage the salt into the scalp or the face and avoid the genital area and nipples. Rinse off the salt with a forceful warm shower followed by a brisk icy-cold shower. Stand under the cold shower for as long as you can manage until you are breathing very deeply. Get out of the bath or shower and dry vigorously.

Turkish Baths and Saunas

In the 1950s and 60s many local councils built excellent public baths equipped with steam rooms (often known as Turkish baths), saunas, icy-cold plunge pools and icy-cold showers. Entrance is often reasonably priced and I generally try and get down to my local one once a week. Turkish baths and saunas increase circulation, skin function, respiration and general vitality, as well as stimulating the nervous and hormonal systems and encouraging mental relaxation and sleep. While in a Turkish bath throw basins of cold water over yourself and, in a sauna, come out and take cold showers or plunges into ice-cold water every two to three minutes after perspiration becomes noticeable. Skin brushing either before or after such baths is particularly helpful for stimulating the nervous and hormonal systems and increasing the circulation.

For those with bronchial congestion or sinus problems, a few drops of eucalyptus, peppermint or wintergreen oil mixed with water, which can be dashed over the coals in a sauna, is helpful, but some people find that as it evaporates it makes their eyes sting so take care. In a Turkish bath, use a small cotton cloth soaked in a few drops of one of these oils and hold it to your face. In either instance breathe in deeply through the nose and out through the mouth.

Hand and Foot Baths

These baths are a particularly useful way of getting children to ingest herbal medicine. I have also used them on some of my adult patients with extremely good effects for oedema, kidney problems, leg ulcers and blood poisoning. They work effectively because they encourage absorption into the capillaries in the soles of the feet and palms of the hands, so allowing full absorption of the herbs directly into the blood and lymph systems. This works much more quickly than through the conventional route of the digestive tract.

Mix double-strength unstrained decoctions or infusions of herbs with an equal quantity of freshly boiled water and pour into a large heat-proof enamel, china or glass container. Immerse the feet in the water, which should be bearably hot, for eight minutes exactly. Do this on rising before breakfast. Hand baths should be taken before supper for the same length of time. Continue this topping and tailing cycle for three days, reheating the mixture as you go and then throwing it out so that you can begin again. Take the bath for six days weekly, resting on the seventh day, and preferably detoxifying the body with a fast on this day.

Mustard hand and foot baths work wonders for aching and burning feet and leg cramps and are a preventative measure against chilblains. Add 1 tablespoon of mustard powder to a bucket of hot water and soak up to the knee or elbow in it for 10 minutes. Massage the hands or feet vigorously afterward with equal parts of simple tincture of benzoin and camphor.

Sitz-baths

These can be awkward, but they are often the most rewarding hydrotherapy of all. A sitz-bath increases the circulation of blood and lymph to the pelvic region, removing internal congestion and improving tissue vitality and nutrition.

In health institutions which use hydrotherapy there are often specifically designed sitz-baths which tend to look like two water-filled armchairs facing one another. One is filled with very hot water, the other with icy cold. You sit with your bottom in the hot and feet in the cold for three minutes and then reverse, leaving your feet in the hot for only one to two minutes. Alternate back and forth from hot to cold for three immersions in each temperature, finishing with your bottom in the hot bath. After drying vigorously with a rough towel, you then exercise until sweating is produced. A simple way to do this is to jog up and down on a trampoline. Alternate hot and cold sitz-baths are useful for any disorders of the uterus, ovaries or Fallopian tubes, for prostatitis, constipation and digestive disorders.

It is possible to imitate these baths at home. Use two large plastic tubs or galvanized wash basins (baby baths do very nicely). They need to be big enough to accommodate the bottom easily and hold enough water to cover you from navel to mid-thigh. The hot water temperature should be as warm as the body can comfortably bear and the cold should be very cold (if necessary, melt ice cubes in the cold water). For maximum benefit carry out these baths at least once and sometimes three or four times daily as instructed.

Cold Sitz-baths

A simple way to do this is to fill your bath tub with 6 in (15 cm) of cold water so that when you sit in it the water comes up to your navel. Now climb in, sit down and raise your feet to above the level of the water, resting them on the edge of the bath. If this is tiring you can put an up-ended plastic bucket as a foot rest. Let your knees fall apart and sweep up handfuls of water, vigorously splashing it over the abdomen while you count slowly to 60. A cold sitz-bath is especially useful for bed wetting, impotence, difficulty in conception and any difficulty with the position of the womb. When you get out, wrap yourself in a towel without drying yourself and lie down for at least 10 minutes. If you feel a nice warm glow after this, gradually increase to a slow count of 180 over 12 sessions or more, so that eventually you are sitting in a bath for up to three minutes at any one time.

Hot Sitz-baths

These are conducted in exactly the same way as cold sitz-baths but the duration can be longer, anything from 3 up to 10 minutes. It is important to take the bath as hot as you can manage it without scalding yourself. It is useful to treat colic and any kind of muscle spasm in the abdomen, lower back pain, haemorrhoids and intestinal disturbances.

Anyone with rectal pain which is so bad that sitting in a hot bath is unbearable should fold two towels into quarters and place them one under each buttock. This will help to turn a hot sitz-bath into a more enjoyable experience and is a particularly useful way of treating haemorrhoids externally (see page 168).

A Sitz-bath Substitute

Stand with your back to the shower so that the warm water is aimed at your lower back only. Now bend forward into the shower, parting your legs so the water runs down between the buttocks, and gradually increase the temperature to the hottest you can manage. Now turn the shower to cold and have it running forcefully over you while you count up to 40. Having mastered this, try to get to count up to 80. When you have finished, dry vigorously with a rough towel and exercise until sweating is produced.

Hot/Cold Shower Routine

This is an easy and very beneficial routine that I put nearly all of my clients through. The hot/cold shower routine stimulates all the body functions, but particularly the adrenal and other endocrine glands, and rejuvenates them. It is also an unbeatable way of revitalizing skin activity and improving the circulation.

Having thoroughly done a dry brush massage (see page 87) take a warm shower for three minutes, if necessary using a natural soap to clean any parts you feel are really dirty. Rinse the soap off well and then switch to the coldest water you can for up to 20 seconds. Switch back to hot water for 2–3 minutes and repeat this seven times so that in all the shower lasts for slightly less than 20 minutes. If there is a particular area in your body which is affected by illness, pay special attention to this area, massaging it vigorously while under both hot and cold. After the hot/cold shower routine, warm yourself up by rubbing down with a coarse bath towel.

Cold Shower Treatment

A cold shower treatment is like a tonic, exerting both rejuvenative and healing effects on the entire system by stimulating the circulation and increasing muscle tone and nerve force. It stimulates the entire glandular system, improving digestion, and speeds up general metabolism. It also increases resistance to infections and colds if used regularly. It has a powerful influence on the central nervous system, on the brain and on every organ in the body. It actually increases the blood count and has an electromagnetic effect on the body, stimulating the flow of life energies and increasing the intake of oxygen to a remarkable degree.

Set your cold shower to the most forceful flow possible because the harder the stream the greater the therapeutic value of the shower. Stand under it and let the forceful stream pound over your entire body for as long as you can manage, but 10 minutes minimum. If it is too tiring to stand up for this time place a plastic stool or chair in the shower. Benedict Lust, a famous nature-cure pioneer, used to administer this to his patients for up to 10 or 12 hours at a time while they were lying on a plastic cot, turning them over on the cot and exposing every part of their body to the forceful stream.

GARGLES

For maximum effect use these as hot as possible. They can be made from infusions, decoctions and tinctures; salt water is effective in relieving sore mouths and throats, providing you do not swallow it. Salt gargle is particularly effective for those unfortunate enough to be stung in the throat.

A few drops of tincture of myrrh in half a cup of hot water is good for mouth ulcers and a double-strength infusion of sage leaves with a teaspoon of cider vinegar added to each cup is excellent for sore throats, including laryngitis. A decoction of ginger root tea with one teaspoon of cider vinegar, two teaspoons of honey, a teaspoon of garlic oil and a generous pinch of cayenne is a delicious mixture to gargle with and then swallow to soothe bacterial throat infections. Tonsillitis can be helped by gargling with a half teaspoon of tea-tree oil diluted in warm water, but spit it out; the pain can quickly be reduced by spraying neat echinacea tincture straight down the back of the throat.

EYE BATHS

These should be made with very gentle herbs like marigold, raspberry leaves, eyebright and cornflower. Brew your herbs freshly, straining them meticulously several times through coffee filter papers.

Always wash out both eyes, with a fresh mixture for each eye, even if only one is affected. Use a sterilized eye bath and change the wash each day. Alternatively, you can apply warm compresses to the eye and keep changing them as they cool. Close your eyes while using compresses. You can also add drops of tincture, usually five to an eye bath of freshly boiled water is about the right dose. By adding the tincture to the hot water the alcohol in it is then rapidly evaporated so it doesn't sting the eye so much, but obviously the water must be allowed to cool to barely lukewarm before being used on the eyes.

VAGINAL DOUCHES

Douches reduce the instance of non-specific vaginitis, relieve painful periods and are essential after the use of vaginal ovules or boluses. These are a very active form of treatment so only use mild herbs, well strained, at body temperature unless otherwise directed and never take more than two douches daily. Even this is only permissible when trying to contain infections. Stop douching as soon as the infection clears otherwise the delicate balance of natural bacteria in the vagina will be altered. The addition of a tablespoon of cider vinegar or a teaspoon of fresh strained lemon juice to every 2 pints (1.1 litres) of herbal infusion or decoction will help to maintain the pH balance.

Your douche kit needs to be kept scrupulously clean. Don't share it with anyone else. Make an infusion or decoction (depending on the herb chosen) and strain through coffee filter paper. Allow it to cool to body temperature. Hang the douche bag (the ones I sell in my own clinic have a strong hook attachment) on the wall over the bath, about 2 ft (60 cm) above the hips. Climb into the bath and lie down. (It helps to warm the bath up first by running hot water around it and then letting it drain out.) Insert the nozzle gently into the vagina so that it actually touches the cervix (which will feel a little like touching your nose with a piece of plastic) and lie back. Now release the closed tap, slowly allowing the herb tea to flow into the vagina. Then using both hands feel the vaginal opening around the nozzle so that the vagina literally becomes flooded. If you do this correctly you will feel a slight sensation of pressure as the vagina expands to accommodate the fluid. When not sexually aroused the vagina is a bit like a squashed corrugated toilet roll, hence the feeling of expansion once filled with fluid. When it feels full, shut the tap with one hand, releasing your hold with the other, and allow your vagina to drain. If you do it correctly the liquid will be rapidly expelled with a big swoosh. Now repeat the whole procedure until all the tea is used up.

Douching while sitting upright on a toilet or bidet is useless because so little actually gets to bathe the vaginal walls before seeping out. Don't bother with it.

Pregnant women should never douche. You should also avoid douching for at least four weeks following delivery.

ENEMAS

These are used to treat nervous complaints, pains and fevers, to cleanse the bowel and stimulate the detoxification of the liver, spleen, kidneys and lymph, and to carry nourishment into the body. Most women who have experienced an enema have usually done so just before childbirth, in an atmosphere of fear and discomfort. Often soapy water was used and this induces violent and painful peristalsis as well as wiping out all the benign bacteria from the colon. I am not, therefore, surprised when I mention enemas, particularly to women, that most of them get very apprehensive. (Enemas are no longer routine before childbirth.)

Let me reassure you: an enema is really easy and comfortable to administer if done correctly. Give yourself plenty of time and privacy and lay everything out in advance because the more relaxed you are, the easier the whole process is.

Contrary to popular fantasy, enemas do not make a mess. Your anal sphincter will hold the liquid in the colon until you decide to release it. Initially the stimulus the enema fluid gives the bowel may make you want to rush straight to the toilet and release it, but you will acquire more self-control with practice and persistence.

Taking an enema is perfectly logical. No sensible person would attempt to unblock a drain from the top end of the waste pipe. Using the same analogy, a blocked colon needs to be relieved from the bottom end. In the event of a fever an enema is the quickest way to relieve the bowel of toxic waste. If you are so weak that you cannot eat, an enema of spirulina or slippery elm will supply some nourishment.

How to Take an Enema

You will need:

- Three and a half pints (2 litres) of a herbal decoction or infusion made with filtered water (cool enemas are used for cleansing and warm ones for treating nervousness and spasms).
- An enema kit (see Resources Directory, page 235).
- Olive oil, Vaseline, or KY jelly.
- A large bath towel or a piece of plastic sheeting.

1 Fill up the enema bag with your chosen infusion or decoction at the right temperature and hang it from a hook in the bathroom at shoulder height.
2 Lubricate the tip well with Vaseline, olive oil or KY jelly.
3 Lie down on your right side with your knees tucked up to your chest and gently push the lubricated tip of the enema tube into the rectum. (Don't worry – it won't slip in too far because it is joined to the kit with a tap which acts as a barrier.)
4 Release the tap and allow the liquid to flow slowly into the rectum. If the liquid encounters a block of impacted faeces you will feel marked internal pressure so turn off the tap, and massage the area in an anti-clockwise direction.

5 When you are halfway through the mixture – you will know this by keeping your eye on your bag suspended from your hook – carefully roll over on to your back with your knees bent and place the soles of your feet flat on the towel or plastic sheet beneath you. When the enema pack is emptied of its contents turn off the tap and remove the nozzle tip.

6 Carefully stand up and wrap yourself in a bath towel then go and lie down on your bed with your bottom raised on some pillows. If you are nervous about spilling any of the enema mixture on to your bed, cover the bed first with a plastic sheet.

7 Retain the enema for 20 minutes if you can. Get up and release while sitting on the toilet.

Note: Enemas should never be relied upon in place of a proper bowel movement, nor should they be abused by over-use.

HERBAL OILS

These are easily obtainable from health-food shops and your local medical herbalist. Garlic oil, borage oil and evening primrose oil can be bought in capsules, although garlic oil is extremely easy to make at home. Cover 4 oz (115g) of fresh garlic with 1 pt (575 ml) of virgin olive or almond oil and liquidize at high speed. Add a tablespoon of cider vinegar to assist the breaking up of the cellulose in the garlic. Pour this mixture into a glass jar, leaving a gap at the top so that the contents can be shaken vigorously. Ideally the jar should be placed outside in strong sunlight embedded in fine sand which attracts and holds the heat for hours after the sun has disappeared. (You may need to store it in the airing cupboard if it is not warm outside.) Bring the jar in at night. Shake again and store it in the airing cupboard until the morning. Keep this routine up for two weeks from the new moon to the full moon, then strain the oil through muslin initially, then coffee filter paper. Bottle the resulting strained oil in dark glass and label.

This process can be speeded up by using artificial heat but I have never found the results as good. Place the jar in a pan of boiling water and keep the water just below boiling point for two hours. Top up the water as needed. This will need more or less constant attention. Strain and bottle when cool. Garlic oil is wonderful for any kind of internal infection and for earache and any sort of external sepsis.

I have made St John's wort oil using the yellow flowers, which is very effective for burns. It comes out a glorious rich ruby red and is also part of my formulation for a deep-heat treatment oil for pulled muscles.

When buying an essential oil always dilute it before applying it to the skin. Essential oil should not be taken internally except under the supervision of a medical herbalist. Do not get undiluted essential oils anywhere near mucous membranes as they will sting.

OINTMENTS

These are easy to obtain from your local health-food shop and local medical herbalist. They are particularly useful for their protective and emollient effects and are usually made with herbal oil and beeswax or cocoa butter. Ointments are good for dry cracked skin. They need to be applied generously and rubbed in thoroughly.

If you want to have a go at making your own ointments, it is not too difficult. Use 1 pt (575 ml) herbal oil to 2 oz (55 g) melted beeswax or cocoa butter, beating vigorously while the mixture cools and thickens. Add essential oils when the mixture has cooled considerably, but before it begins to set. Beeswax gives a stiff pasty consistency while cocoa butter gives a rich oily one.

CREAMS

Creams are better than ointments for treating sore, chapped skin and protecting and moisturizing healthy skin because they are lighter and more easily absorbed. Their moisturizing effect is enhanced if you spray the skin first with flower water or diluted cider vinegar.

It is possible to make your own creams in the same way as you would make an ointment but while emulsifying you also add water, flower water or cider vinegar. These are very tricky to make at home to the right kind of consistency and there are so many excellent ones on the market it is probably better that you buy them, as long as you are sure that all the ingredients are natural.

PESSARIES: OVULES AND BOLUSES

A pessary, sometimes known as an ovule or a bolus, is simply an internal poultice. Pessaries can be used locally to relieve irritation, itching and soreness. Vaginally they will help to relieve chronic reproductive conditions and discharges. The ovule or bolus also influences conditions held deep in the tissues such as tumours, cysts, inflammation, sores and cervical dysplasia (growth abnormality), sending the nutrients to heal the affected area accurately. This is possible because the herbs are absorbed into the mucous membranes and spread through the capillary blood circulation and lymph into the pelvis. If it is supported with herbal nutrients taken internally, total healing should be possible.

Pessaries are made by adding to gently warmed cocoa butter enough finely powdered herbs to form a doughy paste. A vaginal ovule or bolus should be shaped into a sausage the size of a regular tampon with the ends slightly softened and rounded. A pessary should resemble your little finger in size and if it is being used to treat the colon, not only the rectum, it should be at least 2 in (5 cm) long and two should be inserted one behind the other. The best way to roll out the paste is on an oiled marble slab or inside a plastic bag. The pessaries or ovules can then be left overnight on a flat surface in the refrigerator to harden and then stored into sealed plastic bags, each pessary or ovule wrapped in greaseproof paper.

Once unwrapped, the pessary or ovule should be inserted as deeply as possible into the rectum or as high into the vagina as possible just before bed. The body's own heat will then gently melt the cocoa butter and release the herb. Bedlinen should be protected with an old towel and you should wear cotton knickers with a press-on sanitary towel. Alternatively, you can insert half a tampon or a natural sponge to hold a vaginal ovule in place. Rinse the anus or the vagina well the next morning, preferably in a warm followed by a cold sitz-bath. A new pessary should be inserted after every bowel movement, a new ovule or bolus on the evening of every second day. To prevent it coming out while having a bowel movement, insert your finger into the vagina to keep it in place. You should douche on alternate evenings (not the evenings on which you insert an ovule) resting from both douching and the ovules or pessaries on the seventh day.

Often patients say that a pessary has disappeared and wonder how that is possible. It is simply because the body will absorb as much of the herb as necessary and reject the rest, but if it is very much in need of the entire content, all of it will disappear. Sometimes the ovule comes out looking more or less unused and this may be a sign that the treatment is coming to an end and the ovule is no longer needed by the body.

INTERNAL HERBAL TREATMENTS

There are almost as many ways to administer herbs internally as there are externally and these include those based on water, alcohol, sugar, honey and glycerine, all preparations in which the herb is used fresh or in its dried finely powdered form.

HERBAL TEAS

To prepare a herbal tea follow the instructions on page 42 for water-based preparations but avoid powdered herbs which quickly turn into a muddy and unappetizing soup. Keep a teapot especially for your medicinal tea. Your ordinary teapot will tend to get stained with tannin and if you brew an iron-rich tea like yellow dock in such a pot the iron from the herb and the tannic acid from the staining will bond to form tannate of iron, a very strong styptic (an agent that is extremely stringent and contracts tissues, specifically a haemostatic agent which stops bleeding by contracting the blood); this can induce acute constipation and digestive problems.

Always use boiled, filtered water (see page 42).

The quantities of a medicinal tea are always the same unless otherwise specified. These are 1 oz (30 g) to 1 pt (575 ml) of water. The usual dosage is one breakfast-size cup of the strained herbal tea with every meal. Many medicinal herbal teas drunk at this strength taste strong and somewhat unpalatable so can be sweetened with honey, maple syrup, date sugar, liquorice or a dash of apple or grape juice or even grape sugar, but there are certain instances when a tea should not be sweetened: this is mentioned in treatments for specific conditions, such as hypoglycaemia (see page 177). Decoctions are particularly strong tasting and so may need this additional help. If a tea is specifically designed to act on the digestive system, particularly the stomach, liver or pancreas, it may be necessary to drink it without any masking with sweet additions. Teas can be drunk hot as well as cold. Some people find cold decoctions more palatable than hot ones, however hot teas are more stimulating and will act more quickly on the body.

ALCOHOL-BASED PREPARATIONS

These are made in exactly the same way as tinctures are made for external use (see page 43). If you are teetotal and cannot face the thought of alcohol, even for medicinal purposes, or fear your children may be in need of frequent medication with tinctures, simply add the tincture to a little freshly boiled water which will evaporate most of the alcohol out of it. In many instances the use of alcohol to extract a specific property from a herb is essential.

The actual amount of alcohol per dosage is so small that there is more in some commercial mouthwashes than in a herbal tincture. Herbal tinctures are perfectly safe, even for those healing themselves of alcoholism. The dosage for tinctures is generally 1 teaspoon or 15 drops in a cup of water three times a day with meals, but in chronic conditions (such as a diseased heart) I will administer 500 drops of hawthorn tincture daily to a patient and in some acute conditions such as infection I will use 360 drops of echinacea per day to clear it up.

GLYCERINE-BASED PREPARATIONS

It is possible to base a tincture on glycerine which treats the digestive tract more gently than its alcoholic counterpart but such tinctures have the disadvantage of not dissolving oily or resinous materials as effectively.

To make a glycerine tincture, mix one part of vegetable-based glycerine with four parts of filtered water so that you make up 1 pt (575 ml) of the mixture in all. Add 4 oz (115 g) of the dried, ground herb and leave it in a well-stoppered container for two weeks, shaking it vigorously at least once daily (twice if you have the time). After two weeks, strain and press or wring the mixture out in a cloth, catching it in a large basin. Coffee filter paper in this instance is not helpful as the glycerine will not pass through it. Put the glycerine tincture in a labelled bottle and cap it tightly.

SYRUPS

These can be a good way of preparing medication for children as the syrup masks the strong taste of the herb. To a strained decoction, trickle in a quarter of its weight in liquid honey slowly over heat. Stir with a wooden spoon until the mixture turns syrupy. You will need to skim off the rising scum from time to time. Alternatively, mix one part of the tincture with the equivalent weight of honey, stirred over a low heat if necessary to amalgamate the two. Decant into a labelled glass bottle. Take 1 tablespoon (15 ml) as needed.

Syrups are an excellent basis for cough mixture and the old-fashioned and delicious California Syrup of Figs is still available in chemists for children's constipation. Syrups are also very pleasant gargles, when diluted in their equivalent volume of hot water. Whether the gargle is spat out or swallowed the child should be encouraged to clean the teeth afterward to minimize the risk of dental caries.

DRIED PREPARATIONS

My favourite way of administering herbs is in their dried, powdered form. This is probably the most potent and effective form of herbal medicine because the whole herb, rather than an extract, is used. In my own clinic, herbs are generally encapsulated in gelatine capsules but I wish I could get more patients to take them simply in their powdered form mixed with a little water because this is the only way that some of the bitter tasting herbs can be effectively utilized: their effectiveness depends on the neurological sensation of bitterness in order to stimulate the digestive tract.

Dried herbs swallowed in this way take longer to be absorbed by the system because they are unprocessed by water or alcohol, but their action is ultimately far more powerful. If you find you cannot take powders in liquid or in capsules because you have difficulty swallowing, or because you have a particularly sensitive digestive system, you can swallow them with a slippery elm drink. Mix the dried herbs with honey or maple syrup or take the tinctures or extracts made from the powders in juice. If you can swallow herbs in their naked powdered form, buy them direct from the suppliers listed in the Resources Directory (page 233). Alternatively, you can powder your own by putting them through a coffee grinder with a very powerful motor. This will not, however, touch some of the very hard roots and barks, which will have to be purchased already powdered; check that they are as fresh as possible.

GELATINE CAPSULES

These are small cylindrical capsules made from animal or vegetable gelatine in which herbs are compressed. All capsules are available in sizes ranging from 00 to 4. The stock size is 0, the correct size for an adult. It is easy to fill capsules. Simply separate them and press both halves firmly into the powdered herbs until each is as full as possible, then close the capsules carefully together so that one side slots into the other.

The normal dosage for size 0 gelatine capsules is two or three to be swallowed at the beginning of each meal with liquid, preferably herbal tea, fruit or vegetable juice. The food that then follows will ensure their complete assimilation and easy digestion.

Should you have difficulty in swallowing capsules but can manage tablets or vice versa, it may be because you are using the same swallowing technique for both. For a tablet or pill, place it in the mouth with a small amount of water and tilt the head backward. You will find that this way you can swallow more readily. Follow with more liquid. This method does not work for a capsule which, because it is lighter than water, will float forward and so be difficult to swallow. Instead tilt the head or upper part of the body forward then the capsules will float backward and be swallowed easily.

PILLS

These are helpful when herbs cannot be finely powdered but can be roughly chopped and for those who do not have the dexterity or patience to fill capsules. Mix 1 oz (30 g) of the herbs with enough firm set honey or moistened slippery elm powder to make a malleable paste. Divide the paste into 100 equal size portions by rolling it into thin sausages, then cut it into pellets and shape it into balls. Roll each ball so that it is smooth and easy to swallow. Store the capsules that you are going to be taking over the next two days in the fridge and deep freeze the rest in a plastic bag until needed. Because there are no preservatives in either the slippery elm and water mixture or the honey mixture they will spoil even if kept chilled in the fridge after two days.

....

Note: Hypoglycaemics, diabetics and anyone with pancreatic malfunction should not use honey or maple syrup, nor should people trying to lose weight.

....

DOSAGE

As a general rule the dose of any herbs should follow the body weight. Doses in this book are for adults weighing 150 lb (68 kg). Bear this in mind and adjust the dose accordingly. I have found in my own clinic that for people who are underweight or highly strung or possibly both, the best way to take herbs is to spread the dose of the herb out on a more continuous basis throughout the day. This way one capsule, for example, can be taken six times a day with juice or food, rather than three times a day.

HERBAL TEAS

One breakfast-size cup with meals three times a day.

POWDERED HERBS

Two or three size 0 capsules before meals three times a day. This is the equivalent of about 1 oz (30 g) a week. This amount can be increased for nutritional or rejuvenative formulations such as the adrenal or nervine formulations in this book. In this instance you can take anything from 4 to 8 oz (115 to 225 g) a month. I also increase the dose if my client is large or very active or actively wants to pursue a dedicated programme of purification and regeneration. In this instance I start off with average amounts and then escalate the dose upward, depending upon results.

CHRONIC MONTHLY DOSE

If my patient has a chronic condition such as arthritis, rheumatism, colitis or nervous exhaustion I may go as high as 3 oz (55 g) of herbs per week or as much as they can take individually. Much depends on digestive capability, food habits, symptoms, age and levels of pain and discomfort. At this dosage my patient would be taking six to nine capsules with each meal.

Bowel formulations should be taken according to individual need. With the Intestinal Corrective Formulation No. 2 (see page 144) start with only one capsule during or just after dinner. It works best when actively mixed with food. The next morning there should be an increase in bowel action and in the amount of faecal matter eliminated; its consistency should also be softer. If no difference is noticed in bowel behaviour that day, or the difference wasn't dramatic, increase the dose to two capsules that night. Continue to increase the dosage every evening by a capsule at a time until there is dramatic difference in the way the bowels work.

There is no limit with this formulation. Most people only need two or three capsules but I have had a few clients who have needed over 30 capsules. I remind them that it has taken years to create a sluggish bowel so they need to be patient with themselves for a few weeks until the therapeutic action is comfortable and well established.

With the Intestinal Corrective Formulation No. 1, I generally prescribe two capsules at the beginning of each meal and then get the client to increase by one capsule a day only, until the requisite bowel movements are achieved.

The Intestinal Corrective Formulation No. 3 can be taken beginning with one heaped teaspoon liquidized into 8 fl oz (250 ml) of juice once daily and escalating up to five or six heaped teaspoons taken in individual doses, a teaspoon at a time, per day.

SYRUPS

One tablespoon between meals three times a day.

TINCTURES

One teaspoon or 15 drops in a little cold or freshly boiled water, allowed to cool, three times a day.

ACCURATE DOSES FOR CHILDREN AND ANIMALS

I used to calculate the correct dose for a child or animal according to age, but have observed over the years that children's sizes vary dramatically so I have now switched to calculating it by weight. This is more accurate because it is a good pointer to how much the metabolism can handle. Simply make a fraction and put the child's weight over 150 lb (68 kg).

Child's Weight 30 lb

$$ie: \frac{30}{150} \text{ lb} = \text{ ⅕th of the adult dose}$$

If a child's weight was 50 lb (22 kg) they would take one-third of the adult dose. A small dog or cat of 10 lb (4.5 kg) would be one-fifteenth of the adult dose, and a large animal like a horse of 1,500 lb (680 kg) would be 10 times the adult dose.

For children who will not swallow herbs under any circumstances, I would recommend mixing the herbs into organic maple syrup. But if you dilute the tincture or the powdered herbs 50%, the child should be given twice as much as the recommended children's dose that you have already worked out. If in doubt, administer herbs to children through the skin by using hand or foot baths or full body baths. This is an extremely safe and effective method of getting herbs into children, but will not work effectively for certain formulations like the bowel tonics.

Generally, over my many years in practice, I have been able to develop wonderful relationships with children by talking to them quietly and intelligently. Much depends on how herbs are presented to a child. A child is generally a mirror reflection of the parent and if a parent has a scary look upon their face when they try and tell a child that a herbal tonic tastes good, the child is certainly intelligent enough to know they are lying. If in doubt always remember love, hugs and kisses go a long way.

STORING FORMULATIONS

Always sterilize containers before use by boiling thoroughly, and screw on sterilized lids or plug uncapped bottles with generous swabs of cottonwool. Corks will need to be boiled first and then sterilized in diluted cider vinegar.

Anything made with vinegar will keep well over a year if stored in firmly stoppered opaque glass bottles and a tincture made with alcohol will keep for up to five years in these conditions. Dried herbs should be thrown away once they have passed their first birthday. Syrups will keep up to five years but should be stored in a refrigerator, tightly covered, preferably with a vacuum seal. Essential oils will keep indefinitely in small opaque glass bottles but air gaps should be eliminated by transferring them into smaller and smaller bottles as they get used up. Poultices and compresses should always be freshly made and cotton or gauze bandages should be well boiled after use, dried and stored in sealed plastic. If they become sticky with ointment and almost unwashable throw them out. Castor oil may need to be washed off with soap, and then boiled to remove it from poultices.

Any herbal preparation which has gone rotten will smell odd, fizz or turn ominous colours: throw it on your compost heap.

WHEN NOT TO ADMINISTER HERBS

The strict rule when using herbs at home is that no herb should ever be taken even in small quantities unless you are personally totally familiar with its properties and any contraindications. For those who have experience in using harmless herbs for bodily correction there is no need to justify their use.

If in doubt ask for professional help.

One of the enormous advantages of herbal medicine as a therapy is that it is completely safe when correctly administered. In general herbs are certainly far safer than orthodox medicines and many still provide the raw materials for today's allopathic remedies. But I have known amateur herbalists run away with the erroneous belief that all herbs are benign and beneficial and consequently administer them in a spirit of cavalier abandon. This is irresponsible and dangerous. Herbs are very potent healing tools and there are many which are poisonous and should not be used at all.

Occasionally, amateur herbalists poison themselves or worse still, someone else, by ingesting poisonous plants. (Many years ago there was an epidemic of hemlock poisoning, the result of enthusiastic students on a 'Food for Free' kick eating what they thought was wild carrot.) You must remember that many plants have not yet had their biochemical qualities, both toxic and therapeutic, fully documented. There are, for example, 200 species of lupin, two species of laburnum and many others which are intensely poisonous even when taken in minute quantities. What constitutes a toxic dose of the normally therapeutic herb depends largely upon the herb. Often the toxic dose may be 300 times the medicinal dose and herbs in this quantity would be extremely difficult to ingest. There are other herbs that have a toxic dose so close to the therapeutic one that any attempt by the amateur at self-medication may end in disaster. Such herbs are listed on pages 63– 70. Please read this section. I have also included warnings specifically about treating pregnant women and children. In general it is best to treat an acute condition without any herbs at all. Instead fast on fruit or vegetable juices. Fasting is the best medicine of all. However, if you are confident about managing fever there are herbs which are useful for accelerating the patient through this stage.

Qualified herbalists know that when two or more herbs are married in one prescription their individual properties react together in such a way that other effects, not normally found when either of the herbs is prescribed separately, are produced. This marvellous internal co-operation between herbs results in the extraordinary situation of two plus two equalling five. So if a formulation is given in this book which includes more than one herb please do not change it unless an alternative is offered. Never alter the dose of any herb.

If at all doubtful about treating children, don't. Seek the advice of a professional.

CONTRAINDICATIONS OF HERBS

This is a check list of herbs that are contraindicated. Read through it carefully before embarking on taking any of the herbal medicines in this book.

ACONITE

There are some 100 species, all containing the deadly poisonous alkaloids aconitine and pseudoaconitine. If these are ingested in anything but the most minute quantities the results are fatal.

Do not use this herb at all.

ALOE JUICE

This is not to be confused with the whole herb aloe vera or with aloe gel, both of which are potent in their action and should never be used internally. Externally a cut leaf of aloe from the living plant rubbed over burns, rashes, psoriasis, insect bites and itching is extremely helpful but if you ingest the whole plant it will cause internal ulceration and piles. However the juice taken internally actually heals internal ulceration (see Resources Directory).

Normally the dried sap of either Curaçao, Barbados or Cape aloe is used internally, but needs to be mixed with herbs to counteract the griping effect it has on the bowel.

It should never be used by pregnant women.

BELLADONNA

This should only be used by qualified medical herbalists as it is part of the Solanaceae family and one of the better known plant poisons.

BROOM

This should not be used if there is high blood pressure.

It should not be used during pregnancy.

BUTTERCUP

The sap is extremely dangerous taken orally.

CAMOMILE

People often think of this as the gentlest of herbs but over-strong infusions can cause nausea. Go cautiously at first and see how it suits you.

CAYENNE PEPPER

Always take cayenne pepper uncooked. It can cause burning on defecation and this will be helped by mixing it half and half with slippery elm.

CELERY

The problem here is that the seeds are often dressed with a poisonous fungicide so buy organic celery if you possibly can.

Celery is a uterine stimulant and so should be avoided during pregnancy.

CLOVER

Some varieties of white or Dutch clover contain hydrocyanic acid which can poison the digestive system. Ensure that you use red clover only. If using clover externally on the skin it is advisable to mix it into a carrier base such as slippery elm or marshmallow as prolonged contact externally can cause burning and soreness.

COLTSFOOT

Both *Patasites* spp. and *Tussilago* spp. contain pyrrolizidine alkaloids. Other plants in this species are not contra-indicated.

It should be strictly avoided during pregnancy.

COOKED SPICES

Most spices if cooked, as in a curry, aggravate. They are much more therapeutic if taken raw.

CRAMP BARK

This relaxes the uterus so should not be used during pregnancy.

FALSE UNICORN

This contains oxytocic agents which promote delivery. However it is one of the most stimulative tonics to the uterus and ovaries and a superb herb for inducing fertility in women. It can be a gastro-intestinal irritant in large doses.

It should not be used during the course of pregnancy except to resolve potential miscarriage problems and during the last six weeks of pregnancy. This should not be attempted by an amateur.

FOXGLOVE

If taken in excess it is deadly so it should not be used by amateurs.

GARLIC

The whole clove eaten raw is very beneficial for high blood pressure but processed garlic in the form of perles or tablets can actually aggravate the condition. The best breath freshener after raw cloves of garlic is undoubtedly to chew a raw clove, that is, clove the spice.

GINSENG

This is best used in chronic diseases where the patient is weak, cold and debilitated.

It should never be given to those with acute hot fevers nor to those suffering from high blood pressure, or to women with menstrual irregularities.

It should not be taken with anything containing caffeine.

For the elderly or for prolonged treatment of debilitation the maximum dose is 800 mg of the dried root daily. The young and active should not take it for more than three weeks without stopping it for at least a fortnight between doses. For short-term use, the maximum dose is 2 g daily in this instance. This advice applies to Asiatic ginseng (*Panax ginseng*) and American ginseng (*Panax quinquefolius*). Siberian ginseng (*Eleutherococcus senticosus*), although a member of the ginseng family, has a different kind of action. Extensively researched in Russia and given to 20 million Russian workers on a regular basis it has been proved to be the best of all the adaptogens. It increases the productivity and learning capacity of the brain and combats fatigue. It modulates stress hormones through the pituitary–adrenal axis, so helping the body to adapt to non-specific stress and supporting adrenal functions. It is excellent for blood-sugar regulation, jetlag, chronic tiredness and increased endurance. A worthwhile herb to take in tincture form whenever you feel under particular stress.

GOLDENSEAL

If this is taken for more than three consecutive months the person may begin to exhibit hypoglycaemic symptoms. Taken over the long term it will stop the assimilation of B vitamins in the digestive tract. However in the short term it is an excellent antibiotic for anyone.

It is not to be used during pregnancy because it contracts the uterus. It should not be used by diabetics because it lowers blood sugar levels.

GREATER CELANDINE

This has been called both the best and most wicked of herbs and in large doses it is extremely poisonous. Its sale is restricted to medical herbalists only.

GROUNDSEL

Excessive doses over short periods of time may cause cirrhosis of the liver.

HAWTHORN BERRIES

These are not to be used if you have low blood pressure.

HEART'S EASE

Excessive doses can cause a cardiac reaction. Take this under the supervision of a medical herbalist.

HEMLOCK

Most people are familiar with the fact that this is poisonous. Also avoid water hemlock which is equally fatal.

HOLLY

The leaves are sometimes used to treat rheumatism but the berries are poisonous. Make sure no one nibbles them over Christmas.

HORSETAIL

This should always be used with a demulcent herb to soften its effect. (Slippery elm and marshmallow are excellent demulcents.) Horsetail contains silicic acid, saponins, alkaloids and a poisonous substance called thiaminase, which causes symptoms of toxicity in both humans and animals. Thiaminase poisoning causes a deficiency in vitamin B and can lead to permanent liver damage.

JUNIPER BERRIES

Juniper berries are wonderful for clearing up a brief attack of cystitis but should only be used for this kind of emergency, never for prolonged treatment.

LIME TREE FLOWERS

Always ensure your supplies of these are fresh. Old fermenting leaves and flowers can cause hallucinations.

LIQUORICE

This is best avoided altogether during pregnancy because it may affect hormonal balance and decrease the contraction of the uterus. Large and frequent doses exacerbate high blood pressure because liquorice is a cardiac stimulant with a high proportion of sodium.

LOBELIA

This is only available to qualified medical herbalists.

MISTLETOE

Government authorities in the West are sensitive about this herb, mainly I suspect because of its anti-carcinogenic reputation. The berries also contain large amounts of viscotoxins and so are restricted to use by medical herbalists.

NETTLES

If you use the foliage in its fresh state after midsummer it will become a laxative. The sting goes out of the nettle once it is dried. Pick with rubber gloves.

NUTMEG

Nutmeg is perfectly acceptable to use in small quantities in cooking but in large quantities the poisonous alkaloid, strychnine, can result in fatalities.

It should not be used during pregnancy because it can cause abortion.

PENNYROYAL

The essential oil is an abortifacient and should be avoided by pregnant women. The powdered herbs or leaves made into a tea are much milder and can be used in the last six weeks of pregnancy.

PILEWORT

This should never be ingested fresh or rubbed on to the skin fresh because it causes irritation. Once dried, the toxins in the plant break down making it safe to use.

POKE ROOT

The leaves are extremely poisonous. They contain mitogenic substances (that is, substances that distort cell structure). This should be taken under the guidance of a medical herbalist. Properly administered it is an unbeatable cleanser for the lymph and the blood, and is excellent for chronic catarrh and benign cysts.

RED RASPBERRY LEAF

This contains fragine which strengthens the uterus but cannot promote uterine contractions unless a woman has a genetic background of strong pelvic muscles. Its high iron content makes it one of the favourite herbs during pregnancy but it is best administered with the same quantity of another herb.

RUE

If inhaled in large amounts, this is hallucinogenic.

SAGE

Because it is rich in tannin, sage should not be used for a prolonged period of time since tannin builds up proteins and eventually reduces the absorption of B vitamins, which inhibits iron absorption. Very prolonged use of any astringent herb that contains tannin has been associated with throat and stomach cells becoming cancerous so herbs rich in tannin are all best used only for the short term. These include bayberry bark, blackberry, sarsaparilla and yellow dock, as well as peppermint, cleavers and uva ursi.

Sage contains a toxic ketone as part of its essential oil complex, and if the essential oil is consumed regularly over several months this may be emmenagogic, causing womb spasms and the possibility of abortion. Sage oil is therefore not to be used by pregnant women.

ST JOHN'S WORT

In tea or tincture form taken internally, this can cause skin reddening and soreness in some susceptible individuals. The oil used externally on the skin can cause puffiness and swelling. Avoid sunbathing while using this herb in any of its forms.

SASSAFRAS

The oil is carcinogenic so use the whole herb.

....

Do not use during pregnancy at all and do not take longer than three to four consecutive weeks even if you are not pregnant.

....

SHEPHERD'S PURSE

....

This is not to be taken during pregnancy because it stimulates the uterus and contains neurotransmitter precursors.

....

SQUILL

This can cause drastic diarrhoea and retching, and must be given only by a qualified medical herbalist.

TANSY

....

This should not be used during pregnancy as it stimulates the uterus.

....

TOBACCO

Chewed raw or taken as a tea this can cause vomiting, convulsions or respiratory failure, even in minute doses.

VALERIAN

In the short term this is quick and potent if properly prepared but in the long term it can cause degeneration of the nervous system so its long-term use is not desirable.

VIOLETS

Always use the fresh and not the dried flowers.

WHITE BRYONY

In large doses it is toxic.

YARROW

This is an emmenagogue (a substance that stimulates normal menstrual function) and therefore should not be used in pregnancy.

WARNING ABOUT ESSENTIAL OILS

It takes 7,000 or more flowers to make a single drop of undiluted essential oil, so treat all essential oils with a great deal of respect and caution. This applies to both their internal and external use.

If in any doubt at all consult a qualified medical herbalist or aromatherapist.

POISONING BY PLANTS

Induce vomiting as quickly as possible by the age-old method of sticking fingers down the back of the throat (unless the herb was taken several hours beforehand in which case vomiting is a waste of time).

Keep the patient calm. Panic only increases the speed which any poison will invade the system. Don't clear up any vomit until the doctor has inspected it. Undigested plant material in the vomit can give important clues about the nature of the toxic material swallowed. Do not try to induce the vomiting more than once.

Seek immediate professional help.

HERBS FOR SHORT-TERM USE ONLY

After six weeks, replace goldenseal in any formulation with an alternative herb, the nearest are thyme and garlic. Excessive use of goldenseal over a prolonged period can diminish and even stop vitamin B absorption in the digestive tract because it eats up the favourable intestinal bacteria that influence the production and assimilation of these vitamins. Rest a few weeks before going back on to a formulation with goldenseal in it or before taking goldenseal neat. However, it is an extremely effective antiseptic and antibiotic and taken with other herbs increases the tonic properties for the specific organs that are being treated.

QUALIFIED MEDICAL HERBALISTS

Choosing a competent medical herbalist is tantamount to walking through a therapeutic minefield. There are still some excellent herbalists in practice who have no formal qualification whatsoever, just many years of experience, but these are dwindling in numbers. There is a distressing number who have little or no experience and hide behind a list of weekend certificates that mean absolutely nothing. (For a list of qualifications to look for, including medical herbalists that I have trained over the years, see the Resources Directory.) As in every profession the skill of a medical herbalist will vary. Choose someone who will fit into your lifestyle, but whoever you choose look for, and expect, absolute professionalism. I always think the best way to make a choice is to talk to other patients working with a practitioner you have in mind. If a patient has been going to see a practitioner for the last two years and is not improving there is something wrong. It obviously means that the disease is not being helped. Even those with entrenched illnesses like multiple sclerosis who may need to see a medical herbalist for a long period of time should be experiencing some relief.

Many medical herbalists like to see patients for a yearly check-up on a purely preventative basis. I much prefer to work with people who are basically healthy and want to stay that way rather than those who are on their last legs and have tried every other form of medical help before coming to see me. Choose someone who specializes in one field only. A jack of all trades and master of none will be no good to you. Be prepared to work with someone who will open-mindedly refer you on to another branch of natural healing if necessary. Herbalism is not the panacea of all ills. Neither is acupuncture, homeopathy or osteopathy, although judging by the jealous way they cling to their patients, some practitioners evidently believe so.

CHAPTER 3

PREVENTATIVE MEDICINE

———

Diet alone will not achieve good health. There are other essential psychological and physical factors involved. You need to consider the other aspects of your lifestyle. For example, do you smoke? If you are still oblivious to the dangers read the section on smoking (page 222). Are you a passive smoker? If you sit next to somebody who smokes 30 cigarettes a day in a closed office, or smoke this number of cigarettes in the same room as your children, you or they will be ingesting the equivalent of five cigarettes a day. Do you take illegal drugs? The dangers far outweigh any possible benefit that might result from their use. Any high you achieve will be temporary and the toxic residues left behind horrendous. Try not to take drugs for any reason at all, including medical ones unless they are absolutely essential. There are more ways to ease a headache than dashing to the medical cabinet for an aspirin.

Aspirin produces vitamin losses, particularly of vitamins B and C, in the system. It interferes with the series of chemicals in our bodies called prostaglandins, inhibiting some of them, then raising the temperature of the body. Prostaglandins play a major part in creating inflammation in the body so while aspirins are prescribed for the inflammation of joints (besides headaches), they are also widely used to interfere with blood clotting and are often thought of as blood thinners. In fact it takes longer for bleeding to stop after aspirin has been swallowed, precisely because of the effect it has on platelets, a key component of blood clotting. A single aspirin inactivates all the platelets in the blood for a considerable length of time and only a fraction of an aspirin, about one-tenth, is needed to deactivate all the platelets in circulation in the bloodstream at any one time. These platelets are constantly being replenished by the bone marrow, from which all the blood cells are produced. They survive between 10 and 14 days within the circulatory system and every day we lose 10% of them. The newly released platelets are not affected by a dose of aspirin given the day before but by aspirin taken on the same day, which is precisely why doctors ask patients not to take any aspirin for at least a week before surgery: one aspirin taken close to an operation may result in intra-operative bleeding and increase the likelihood of the patient needing a blood transfusion.

In addition, aspirin is a severe stomach irritant, it can cause temporary infertility as well as loss of hearing and tinnitus and it has been known to cause allergies, swollen lymph nodes, generalized swelling, drops in blood pressure, breathing problems, diarrhoea, nasal polyps and hives. Flu and chickenpox should never be treated by aspirin because such treatment may cause Reye's disease, which can be fatal. The now widespread use of aspirin to prevent strokes is not supported by scientific evidence. All in all, wouldn't you rather try an alternative cure for an headache? Meditate, lie down in a darkened room and have a short nap, have a massage with a few drops of lavender oil, take half a cup of feverfew tea, place some ice cubes on your forehead or a hot water bottle on the back of your neck.

Regular physical exercise is essential in order to maintain good health but have you ever thought about taking regular mental exercise? Good mental health is a prerequisite of physical health. Watching large amounts of television or videos has an almost hypnotic effect on some people, particularly children. In addition, too many people hug the television set by sitting far too close, and so are bathed in the radiation which leaks from every television set. Hours spent in front of the television set will mean exposure to ELFs (extremely low frequencies) and the possibility of disturbed sleep. Of course electrical and magnetic fields surround all electrical conductors, whether giant power lines or the wiring in your house and electrical appliances. EMFs (electro-magnetic frequencies) are made up of electrical fields and magnetic fields and what they create is rather like the static electricity you may feel when you get a shock from walking on a new carpet. Unless you live close to a major power line this isn't a problem because they can be shielded by walls and trees. Magnetic fields generated by electrical current, however, can travel right through walls and cannot be shielded, but only modified by the careful design of wiring and electrical equipment. Hence the growing concern about microwaves, television masts and transmitters. Most transmission could more safely be sent by cable or fibre optics.

EMFs have been linked to depression, heart attacks, suicide, adult cancers and childhood leukaemia, as well as minor problems such as headaches, insomnia and irritability. The fields created by electric blankets and heated water beds have been found to increase the likelihood of miscarriages among pregnant women.

Bearing all this in mind it is sensible to take protective measures – but do keep a sense of proportion. Remember two factors: duration and distance. Viewing a television set from 12 feet (3.7 m) away will considerably reduce the effect of ELFs, but sleeping on an electric blanket which is switched on all night produces unacceptably high levels of ELFs. Microwave ovens and conventional electrical cookers generate large ELFs because of the heavy current they consume. If you can, and you have no respiratory difficulties, cook with gas. For some years now the Russians have banned the construction of buildings within a kilometre of power lines. So if you are considering buying a house near a power line, it might be safer not to.

If you want to keep the mind active, play a board game or intricate card game, study a new subject with concentration, design a dress, or even do a difficult crossword puzzle.

People who set themselves achievable goals in life often have a much more positive attitude and something to live for. All work and no play makes you dull. On the other hand if you continually avoid your responsibilities you will tend to get dragged down with misery and guilt. Stress caused by a sense of failure and self-recrimination is far worse than the stress caused by extra responsibility.

People who live in dirty, untidy environments tend to encourage the same state internally, physically and mentally. It is difficult to feel relaxed and serene in surroundings that are chaotic or dirty. The Chinese have known about the importance of a harmonious and comfortable environment and its study, *feng shui*, for thousands of years. In the West we have only begun to wake up to its importance through our recognition of geopathic stress since the middle of this century.

NATURAL LIVING

All good health is concerned with balance. It is just as important to assimilate efficiently as it is to eliminate. Repairs can only take place in the midst of decay, so nature has to clean out the old debris before she can rebuild good solid foundations. No one facet of health dominates any other. All are equally important.

ASSIMILATION

The famous maxim 'you are what you eat' should be more accurately stated as 'you are what you assimilate'. I have worked with patients who are very conscientious about their diet and eliminate with the precision of a sergeant major but if they are not making full use of that food it is all a waste of time and money. More often I encounter those who fill themselves with inorganic vitamins and minerals until they rattle and are still creeping around half-dead because the substances from which such supplements are made are stressing the body to such an extent that it is unable to assimilate them. Or there may be some organ, gland or system which is damaged, malformed, traumatized or underdeveloped and so unable to function efficiently metabolically without appropriate healing.

CHEWING

Correct digestion begins in the mouth. Saliva is full of ptyalin which helps to break down starch, so if you gulp your food or talk excessively while eating or worse still try and sit down and eat when you are worried or distressed, you won't be able to make full use of it. Try and chew your food patiently until it is a liquid pulp before swallowing it.

STAY CALM

The metabolic process of the body is much more upset by negative feelings such as greed, fear, distress, rage, shock, guilt, anxiety, jealousy, depression and grief than a mouthful or two of 'naughty' food. Emotional equilibrium is the key to digesting food properly. If you are upset, miss the meal. If you are upset but still feel hungry, sip a glass of freshly pressed fruit or vegetable juice slowly swishing it through your mouth and warming it up before swallowing each mouthful. Try never to eat to comfort yourself or to relieve tiredness. Never force other people to eat or put more food on their plates than they ask for. This is a habit which, when taken from childhood into adulthood, can prove very destructive.

It takes four hours to empty the stomach completely. The ideal eating pattern as outlined on page 36 is a light breakfast, a good sustaining lunch and a light evening meal eaten not later than 7–8 p.m. If you are hypoglycaemic you will need to eat little and often. Protein snacks taken every two hours are much more helpful for this condition. By following this pattern you won't tax your body's enzymic systems or its pattern of assimilation and elimination.

DIGESTIVE AID

Equal parts of tinctures of ginger, fennel, peppermint and liquorice will normalize stomach acids helping to remove any excessive acid, prevent wind and mucous congestion and comfort the stomach, intestines, nerves and glands. As an added bonus it tastes good. Take 15 drops in a little water or directly on the tongue as often as needed.

THE PHILOSOPHY OF NATURAL HEALING

'There are three stages through which a person must pass in getting well. They are the eliminative, the transitional and the building stages. The crisis usually occurs during the transitional period, which is the time when the new tissue has matured sufficiently to take on the functions of a more perfect body.'

Dr Bernard Jensen

By following the laws of nature, healing takes place as surely and as naturally as the sun rises and sets. Dr Jensen is now an elderly naturopath living in the United States who has been revered for the superb work he has done over many years at his own healing ranch. He has helped literally thousands of people to heal themselves, some of them of extremely serious illnesses, so his observations come from years of experience. He recently healed himself of pancreatic cancer in his late 80s.

The first stage of healing is to open up the eliminative channels and get rid of any congestion or waste. In my experience an iridology test is perhaps the most valuable way of finding out exactly how your eliminative organs are functioning. I can safely say that nearly 80% of the people who consult me are in some way drowning in their own poisons, a condition that we naturopaths term auto-intoxication, meaning literally self-poisoning.

Most people think that what they see in the toilet is what they ate a couple of meals back but a normal 20th-century diet ensures that a lot gets left behind in the colon that doesn't come out at all. Colonic or rectal cancer, in both men and women, is the most widespread cancer in the Western world. Even the notoriously conservative American Medical Association (AMA) have admitted that the main reason for this is dietary. Hundreds of thousands of people suffer from other disorders of the colon and everyone at some time in their lives has experienced some type of bowel disorder, generally constipation or diarrhoea. The fact that thousands of tons of laxatives and anti-diarrhoea medicines are sold all over the Western world confirms this.

In an average bowel movement there may be starches that haven't been digested properly by pancreatic secretion. Drugs and barium meals, as well as catarrh-forming foods like dairy products, sugar and eggs, get pasted on to the sides of the colon turning into encrusted mucus the weight of which forces the wall of the colon outward to form diverticular pockets. It is now estimated that more than 80% of men and women over the age of 60 have diverticular pockets in their colon. In some people this encrusted waste can cause the colon to weigh as much as 40 lb (18 kg) and to balloon out from the customary 4 in (10 cm) to as much as 9 in (23 cm).

The fact is that our modern lifestyles have wreaked havoc with our colons. You should have a bowel movement for every meal you eat, therefore if you eat three meals a day, you should have three reasonably copious bowel movements a day. Constipation is the hub of the mechanism in the disease process. The heart of the problem lies in the passage of toxins and micro-organisms through the intestinal wall into the body in general causing an endless array of disturbances. When the body absorbs poison from the decaying waste in the colon every other organ has to bathe in this poison. Meat, fish and eggs provide the most harmful metabolites which, on entering the bloodstream, create a toxic blow for the cells throughout the body, in particular the liver and kidneys. Auto-intoxication causes fatigue, poor concentration, irritability, insomnia, muscular aches, headaches, poor skin and bad breath and can lead to all the degenerative diseases including cancer. It has been observed that the populations with a high instance of colonic and rectal cancer consume diets containing less fibre, grains, vegetables, fruits, nuts and seeds and more animal and protein fat and refined carbohydrates than populations with a low instance of the disease. Bouts of diarrhoea are common in sufferers of constipation, and caused when a substance irritates the colon so badly that peristalsis goes into overdrive in an attempt to expel it. The build-up of faecal matter trapped in the colon becomes so great that this induces a state of continuous peristalsis resulting in chronic diarrhoea.

CONSTIPATION

FACTOR	CAUSES OF CONSTIPATION	PROMOTES GOOD COLON ELIMINATION
Food	Meat and all animal products, eggs, dairy products and any highly refined food.	Fruits, vegetables, grains, seeds, nuts. Live food creates life. When you start to eat it, you will actually feel new activity in your bowel.
Liquid	Not enough liquid, dehydrated foods.	Drink one gallon (4.5 litres) of liquid every day, in the form of water, herbal teas and fruit and vegetable juices.
Movement	Sedentary lifestyle with a lot of sitting or lying down.	All movement, especially deep breathing and abdominal exercise. Even walking can work wonders.
Emotional	Fear, or negativity, holding on to problems, holding on to old, useless material possessions.	Courage, letting go of people and things, opening up your mind, being an open, aware and loving person.
Drugs	Any drugs which sedate or are narcotic with opiate derivations such as codeine.	Digestive, stimulating and cathartic herbs.
Intestinal flora	Antibiotic drugs, extremely hot food, essential oils, loud noises (over 72 decibels), X-rays, sudden violent changes in weather, bottlefeeding as a baby.	Fermented nuts, seeds, grains and vegetables such as sauerkraut, positive ions, breastfeeding from birth, garlic.
Toilet	Sitting upright on a Western-style toilet necessitates pushing down against the rectum and positively encourages haemorrhoids.	Squatting with your feet elevated on a box or pile of magazines to within 6 in (15 cm) of the toilet seat with your knees spread and your elbows resting on them is the ideal way to take a bowel movement, and this position relieves the bearing down on rectal muscles.

A GOOD BOWEL MOVEMENT

Many of my patients have libraries in their bathrooms. If you have time to read while sitting on the toilet, you have constipation.

Having a bowel movement should be easy, comfortable and quick. When you feel the urge, you should be able to evacuate your bowels in a few minutes and be finished, without straining, squeezing or grunting. Every bowel movement should be soft and mushy like cottage cheese, slightly gaseous and should crumble and break up as it reaches the water on the surface of the toilet. If it is well formed or any harder or dryer than this you are constipated (see also Constipation, page 138). Remember, ideally you should be having a bowel movement for every meal you eat, but in no case, even when fasting, should you have less than two a day.

A properly functioning bowel means better food assimilation, increased vitality and better absorption of nutrients and it often reduces the desire to eat as much food. With chronic constipation only 10% of the food eaten is utilized. Most laxatives are poisonous and merely irritate the bowel, doing nothing to remove the encrusted mucus. If laxatives are used regularly the colon becomes addicted to them and in time grows weaker from over-stimulation and irritation so that the dosage has to be increased.

The triangle of environmental, emotional and biological or physical stress which is the basis of many illnesses applies particularly to the bowel. People are often reluctant to let go of faecal matter simply because they are so uptight by nature. In this case simple relaxants such as skullcap or valerian are often helpful in relaxing the bowel enough to allow it to do its work naturally.

EXERCISE

Exercise is a vital factor in good bowel health. In order to encourage peristalsis, use your legs. Their movement improves circulation and lung capacity, and strengthens the abdominal muscles, thereby stimulating the peristaltic action of the bowel.

FRIENDLY BACTERIA

Every colon holds 3 to 4 lb (1.4 to 1.8 kg) of resident bacteria as indigenous flora. This is made up of 300 to 400 different species of bacteria whose activities affect our metabolism, physiology and biochemistry in ways that are both beneficial and harmful.

These micro-organisms are either indigenous or transient. The former colonize particular ecological niches in the intestinal tract by adhering to the mucosal epitheliums; the latter are ingested in food and drink and are constantly in transit from the mouth to the anus. Together they make up nearly 40% of the whole weight of our faecal matter.

The bacterioids, together with coliform bacilli and E. coli, are the putrefactive bacteria responsible for the decaying matter in the colon. They enjoy a diet full of protein and fat which accelerates the output of undesirable metabolites like bile salts, urea, phenols, ammonia and other dietary degradation products which are all potentially harmful, doubly so if there is already constipation or a malfunctioning liver present. A high population of harmful bacteria is one of the main contributory factors to the development of all sorts of degenerative diseases like ulcerative colitis, diverticulitis, haemorrhoids and colonic cancer. Unfortunately most people have a ratio of 85% of these potentially harmful bacteria to only 15% beneficial bacteria.

The beneficial bacteria produce acetic, lactic and formic acid which lower the pH of the intestine, so preventing the colonization of fungus like *Candida albicans*. When the percentage is better balanced, with 75% of the goodies, peristalsis is stimulated, flushing out toxic bacterial metabolites and waste products in the faeces and so checking putrefactive bacteria.

INTESTINAL FLORA

Certain foods are known to promote benign intestinal flora. These include natural, raw, unsalted sauerkraut, miso soup and fermented grains like rejuvelac, as well as some herbs, especially garlic. Garlic is capable of destroying bacteria that are harmful to us while actually increasing the good bacteria.

The most vicious destroyers of beneficial intestinal flora are antibiotics. Whether we consume them as by-products of the meat or dairy industry or take them for infections, all antibiotics cause enormous quantitive as well as qualitative changes in our intestinal flora, creating a perfect seed bed for pathogenic micro-organisms and actively encouraging the growth of *Candida albicans*. The radiation of the abdomen with gamma rays or X-rays upsets the normal microbial balance of the colon, as do sudden violent changes in the weather and prolonged loud music (above 72 decibels).

STRESS

The profound effect of stress on intestinal ecology is interesting. It doesn't matter what the source of the stress is; the stress response stimulates the release of adrenalin and cortisol as the body alerts itself for 'fight or flight'. These hormones then induce a number of physiological changes, including the drying up of oral and gastric secretions, the retention of sodium chloride and the acceleration of potassium excretion and raised blood sugar. All these reactions cumulatively alter the intestinal habitat, decreasing the micro-organic goodies and increasing the baddies. When you consider how much routine stress you are exposed to – bright lights, atmospheric pressure, noise, crowds, long journeys – and how much more is self-generated – from fatigue, anger, anxiety, pain and fear – it really makes you appreciate just how hard it is to generate the right sort of balance.

CORRECTIVE FORMULAS

The intestinal corrective formulas originally designed by Dr Christopher, the world-famous American herbalist, and by Richard Schulze are intended to help proper bowel function and aid elimination (see pages 142, 144 and 152).

THE LIVER

The main function of the liver is to maintain the body's dynamic balance by preparing fats, carbohydrates and protein for its use, by storing some nutrients, by manufacturing enzymes, bile, antibodies and the specific proteins needed for blood clotting and by maintaining the proper blood levels of glycogen, amino acids, hormones and vitamins, as well as neutralizing any poisons which enter the bloodstream.

Our livers have a particularly hard task today because they are inundated with chemicals, the result of environmental poisoning or totally synthetic food. Indeed we eat substances which are so heavily processed that they can no longer be recognized as food. Even some brands of wholemeal brown bread contain as many as eight additives.

If your liver is ailing you may have feelings of heaviness or discomfort in the area of the lower margin of the ribs on your right side, coupled with a feeling of general sluggishness and tiredness for no reason. Indigestion with flatulence may go on for years, as may alternating constipation and diarrhoea. The tongue is often thickly coated, white or yellow, and bad breath may be a problem.

Eating only natural healthy foods and living in an environmentally clean atmosphere will delight your long-suffering liver. Stressed livers particularly hate all processed, fried and fatty foods, especially dairy products and deep-fried food. They need plenty of vitamins A and D and calcium to assist them to maintain healthy internal mucosae. Alcohol should be taken in moderation: leave at least three days a week alcohol free. Livers particularly benefit from a daily ingestion of lecithin granules (available in health-food stores) which can be sprinkled into any soup or bowl of porridge. They also like plenty of garlic, ginger, onions, vegetables from the mustard family and lemons.

A SPRING CLEAN FOR THE LIVER

Spring is a particularly appropriate time to do a liver cleanse because the body is just emerging from a winter of heavy fatty congestive foods and not enough exercise. Liver flushes are an excellent way of stimulating the elimination of waste from the body by opening and cooling the liver and increasing the bile flow, so improving overall liver function. They also help to purify the blood and the lymph. My favourite liver flush is as follows.

LIVER FLUSH

Take one (building up to three) cloves of garlic and 1 in (25 mm) of peeled fresh ginger. Liquidize them at high speed in 8 fl oz (250 ml) of juice, with a thinly pared and sliced fresh lemon. As you liquidize add 1 to 4 tablespoons of flax seed or organic olive oil. The juice you choose can be a combination of freshly squeezed citrus juices, apple, carrot or carrot and beetroot. Garlic and ginger have excellent liver protective qualities and garlic particularly provides important sulphur compounds that the liver needs to build enzymes.

LIVER TONIC

Equal parts of tincture of:
milk thistle
dandelion
Oregon grape
gentian
wormwood
black walnut
ginger
garlic
fennel.
Add 70 drops of this to the liver flush while liquidizing and take a further 70 drops in water four more times after eating for a week.

LIVER TONIC

The herbs in the liver tonic tincture are famous for their ability to stimulate, cleanse and protect the liver and gall bladder and rid the body of parasites. Milk thistle has certain chemicals that bind and coat liver cells not only healing previous damage but also protecting the liver from future damage. The Oregon grape, gentian, wormwood and dandelion stimulate digestion, helping the liver to excrete more bile which in turn cleans both the liver and gall bladder. This is a particularly useful formulation for anyone who has had constipation, eaten large amounts of animal foods including dairy products throughout their life or drunk alcohol, tea or coffee or chocolate in large quantities. It is also particularly recommended for high cholesterol, or a family history of liver or gall bladder problems.

This formulation works best if done simultaneously with a bowel cleanse. You may keep it up for between one and four weeks in the spring, while adhering to a light diet and fasting on the seventh day on carrot and beetroot juice or carrot and apple juice. You may notice your faeces will produce a little green colouring during the cleanse or, better still, you may notice some parasites coming out of your bowel movements because there are a number of anti-parasitical herbs in the formulation. Remember a 1 in (25 mm) cube of beef can contain over 1,000 parasite larvae just waiting to hatch in your body, and as much as 65% of fresh fish may have toxic levels of bacteria and parasites.

Follow any liver flush with one or two cups of piping hot detox tea.

DETOX TEA

Equal parts of:
roasted chicory
roasted dandelion root
liquorice root
ginger
coriander seeds
orange peel
hawthorn berries
cinnamon sticks
carob pods
fennel seeds
clove buds
black peppercorns
parsley
juniper
uva ursi
horsetail.

To make this tea as effective as possible put two tablespoons into 1 pt (575 ml) of pure water allowing the tea to steep in cold water overnight. In the morning heat to a boil while tightly covered, then simmer for 15 minutes. Strain out the herbs but do not discard them. Drink two cups of the liquid as hot as possible and then put the herbs back into the pot. Add a tablespoon of fresh herbs and a further 1 pt (575 ml) of pure water. Let it sit overnight and repeat the whole process again. Keep adding new herbs from the old ones for three days, then discard all the herbs and start again.

DETOX TEA

This tea is based on an old East Indian digestive tea formulation known as yogi spiced tea. It is stimulating to the digestion, soothes the stomach, and is mildly cleansing for the blood, skin, liver and gall bladder. It also flushes out the bile and fats that the liver flush has purged out of the liver and gall bladder, and is a mild diuretic and disinfectant to the kidneys and bladder – it may make you urinate a little more within an hour after ingestion. Best of all it is an excellent coffee replacement and tastes good. It increases the circulation but has no caffeine and will help you to get off the coffee and tea habit.

Do not eat or drink anything for one hour after your liver flush. If possible use the time to lie down with a castor oil poultice over your liver. When the hour is over drink 8 fl oz (250 ml) of prune juice. If you make it yourself, soak ten organic prunes in two glasses of water overnight. Liquidize this in the morning but remember to take the pits out first. Prune juice has an extraordinary ability to draw toxins from every part of the body and eliminate them through the bowel which is why bowel movements after prune juice often smell so strange and strong.

MAJOR GALL BLADDER FLUSH

This is recommended only for those who are already experienced with fasting and cleansing and want to remove even more old wastes stored in liver cells and other tissues. It is an extremely strong cleanse but of the hundreds of gall bladder flushes I have supervised I have never seen patients become anything more than nauseated at the very worst. It should not be undertaken without the supervision of a medical herbalist.

This activates the liver and gall bladder even more strongly than the liver flush. By combining it with a three-day juice fast, toxic waste released during fasting will be effectively eliminated during the strong bile flush and enema. People very often eliminate lots of green putty-textured stones and, while I have heard them called gall stones manufactured from cholesterol, I feel they may well be saponified oil.

I have also observed a lot of anger, negativity and frustration purged during the course of a gall bladder flush. And, in groups, people may behave as if they were drunk. Whether this is due to old drug residues being re-experienced as they are eliminated from the body or the result of a systemic hormonal reaction to all that oil doesn't really matter. Either way the gall bladder flush is an extremely powerful and effective cleanse for the liver and gall bladder.

At seven o'clock in the evening of the third day of your juice fast, liquidize 1 pint (575 ml) of organic olive oil with the juice of nine freshly squeezed lemons and take five tablespoons every 15 minutes. If you find yourself vomiting up any olive oil, continue to take the remainder but do not go back to the beginning. Sucking an ice cube or sipping a little decocted ginger tea in between doses of oil and lemon juice often helps with nausea.

If you find drinking olive oil in such large quantities truly horrendous, sip it through a straw so that it does not contact the lips but goes right down the back of the tongue and throat easily. Once you have finished drinking the oil go to bed with a warm castor oil compress over the liver and a hot-water bottle. Lie on your right side with your knees tucked up and your hips elevated and stay in this position for at least two hours unless you are actually sitting up to drink the olive oil and lemon juice. Meanwhile distract yourself with some of your favourite music or a good video if you can see it from this angle.

If you need anything else to drink sip only ginger tea or water.

The next morning take a chicory enema or a warm-water enema with the juice of half a lemon squeezed into it. Both will help to stimulate elimination but the chicory one is more effective. People bring me gifts of what they consequently produce in jars and the 'gall stones' range in size from gravel to beans and seeds to lumps the size of golf balls. If stored in a jar they will dissolve within a couple of days. In order to retrieve them (and naturally this is for your own interest only and possibly that of your practitioner) you will need to wash the bowel movements with running water through a sieve so defecate in a potty.

Note: This cleanse should only be done once a year and should always be preceded by at least ten days of the liver flush.

THE KIDNEYS

Any job which ought to be done by the kidneys but which is not will result in impure blood returning to the heart. This is one of the reasons why diuretics are often prescribed for heart problems by allopathic doctors but remember that all chemical diuretics work by irritating the delicate tubules in the kidneys, forcing them to pass water and in doing so leaching potassium from the body, so much so that synthetic potassium has to be given in its place.

Herbal diuretics have in-built safety because they contain potassium and the various complex nutrients needed to maintain an efficient input and output. They raise both potassium and sodium levels so that the cellular pump-action improves both ways. For example, celery is high in sodium with a touch of potassium while dandelion is high in potassium with a little sodium.

Healthy kidneys need to be constantly flushed out so drink lots of pure water and potassium-rich broth made from tough outer green leaves of vegetables and potato skins (for recipe see page 31). Cut out tea, coffee, cocoa, salt and alcohol completely and drink plenty of fruit and vegetable juices. Follow a diet which is high in fresh fruit and vegetables and keep it free as far as possible from processed foods. Strawberries are especially useful for dispelling uric acid.

NEVER IGNORE A FULL BLADDER

I am amazed how seldom many of my patients urinate, often only two or three times a day. The contents of the bladder are subjected to chemical change if harboured too long so by holding on, the lining of the bladder gets intensely irritable. A full bladder will press down on all the pelvic organs, especially the lower bowel and reproductive organs, and aggravate the possibility of prolapse.

If we are eliminating efficiently we should lose at least 1 gallon (4.5 litres) of water every day through the skin, the kidneys and other eliminative organs. If your kidneys are malfunctioning evidence of water retention includes puffy ankles, swollen fingers and feet which spill over the sides of your shoes. Waterlogged kidneys are evident by dark circles and bagginess under the eyes.

Barley water is an ideal drink to soothe and cleanse the kidneys and maintain them in peak condition. It has the added bonuses of strengthening the nails and improving the quality and quantity of the milk of lactating mothers, and helps to relieve asthma because of the hordein it contains.

BARLEY WATER

Pour 1½ pints (850 ml) of water over 1 oz (30 g) of whole-grain barley (pot barley won't do) and boil until the quantity is reduced by half. Add the zest of one lemon and sweeten with a little organic maple syrup, organic honey or apple juice if desired. Drink freely at room temperature. It tastes very pleasant.

KIDNEY FLUSH

On rising add to 16 fl oz (500 ml), escalating to 32 fl oz (900 ml) of pure water (it can be warmed) the juice of a freshly squeezed lime and lemon (if limes are not available, use two lemons). Add a generous pinch of cayenne pepper and if desired organic maple syrup to sweeten. To this add the following mixture.

KIDNEY BLADDER TONIC

Equal parts of:
uva ursi leaves
juniper berries
cornsilk
horsetail
burdock
goldenrod
parsley
in tincture form.
Add 60 drops to the morning drink. This tonic is both diuretic and disinfectant. It works best if you take a further 60 drops four more times during the course of the day in extra liquid and should be used alongside the kidney bladder tea.

KIDNEY BLADDER TEA

Equal parts of:
juniper berries
cornsilk
uva ursi
parsley
dandelion
horsetail
goldenrod
hydrangea root
gravel root
marshmallow root
orange peel
peppermint.
Use leaves or berries in every instance except for the roots and the orange peel. Make as a decoction and drink two cups three times a day. You can keep up this kidney cleanse for a month.

If in the summer you want to do some further kidney cleansing, fast for three days on water melon juice. Include some of the seeds and 1 sq in (6.5 sq cm) of the rind juiced into every 8 fl oz (250 ml) of juice. Known as a water melon flush, this is an extremely effective diuretic. You can also include potassium broth on your three fasting days in copious amounts.

THE SKIN

If your skin is spotty or has a poor texture it may be evidence of a chronically congested bloodstream or bowel. Dr Christopher offered an excellent blood purifying formulation which contains not only blood rebuilders but cleansers and astringent herbs to increase the range and power of the circulation, particularly to those parts of the body which have been deficient (usually the extremities like the hands, head and feet). This formulation also removes cholesterol, kills infection and makes the veins more elastic while strengthening the artery walls so that the herbal nutrients in it will travel through the blood and lymph and be effectively utilized.

DR CHRISTOPHER'S BLOOD PURIFYING FORMULA

> *Equal parts of:*
> *buckthorn bark*
> *burdock root*
> *chaparral*
> *liquorice root*
> *Oregon grape root*
> *peach bark*
> *prickly ash bark*
> *red clover blossom*
> *stillingia.*
> *All herbs should be finely powdered and put into size 0 gelatin capsules. Take three capsules with each meal. If you get diarrhoea, it means that the formulation is working too hard and may also indicate the urgent necessity for bowel and liver purification. Attend to these two and then try to reduce the dose of the blood purifying formula to a comfortable level.*

Regular exercise involving profuse sweating will help the skin. The sweat excreted from such exercise contains more toxic waste than the sweat you flush out during the course of a Turkish bath or sauna. However, these do help too, so don't reject them.

Neither treatment should be taken if you have high blood pressure or are pregnant.

Too many people suffocate their skins with synthetic fabrics. Wear only natural fabrics next to the skin. The healthiest fabric is cotton or failing that linen, silk or wool. Remember the palms of the hands and soles of the feet are particularly richly endowed with sweat glands so never suffocate these areas with non-leather shoes or nylon socks.

I do not recommend the routine use of synthetic soap all over the body. Choose an organic rather than a detergent soap (see Resources Directory) and use only on areas that are particularly sweaty or dirty. Skin brushing will do the rest. Never put anything on your skin that you wouldn't be prepared to eat. A few drops of a herbal essential oil mixed in a carrier base of almond or olive oil and added to bath water will act therapeutically on the skin, as well as moisturizing it. Don't use mineral oil (sometimes sold as baby oil) or products containing it (many commercial cleansing creams do).

Try to avoid synthetic antiperspirants or deodorants because they block the skin's natural cleansing action and destroy the natural bacteria on the skin, upsetting its delicate protective pH balance. (Many also contain aluminium, which is poisonous.) If you smell particularly obnoxious, it is because your body is off-loading toxins through your skin and you need to look at the inside not the outside to remedy the problem. Washing twice daily should keep you smelling sweet. If it doesn't use a natural deodorant (for a supplier see Resources Directory). Alternatively wash more often until your body's purification is complete.

Don't wash your clothes with detergents that contain enzymes. In some people the body's defence mechanism responds to enzymes by launching an assault as if it were attacking an infection and sooner or later you may end up developing a serious form of skin irritation.

SKIN BRUSHING

Because our skin is the largest two-way eliminative organ in our bodies, flushing outward by way of perspiration and absorbing nutrients and vitamins from natural sunshine, it is worth taking special care of. The skin also breathes and absorbs oxygen while exhaling carbon dioxide formed in tissues. The hundreds of thousands of sweat glands which should operate to expel at least 1 lb (450 g) of waste products daily regulate body temperature and act as miniature detoxifying organs working to cleanse the blood and free the system of suffocating poisons.

Help the skin to eliminate daily by dry skin brushing for five minutes followed by the seven times hot/cold shower routine (see page 50).

The benefits of skin brushing must be tried and tested to be believed. You will feel clean, refreshed and much more alert. Skin brushing stimulates the circulation helping to pump the blood down through the veins and up through the arteries, feeding those organs of the body which lie near the surface. It also stimulates the lymph and adrenal glands and, because of the hundreds of nerve endings in the skin, has a powerful rejuvenating effect on the nervous system.

By vigorously skin brushing over the major lymph glands – dumping stations for waste fluids – you can stimulate the expulsion of mucoid lymphatic material or impacted lymph. (This is more commonly known as cellulite.) These lymph glands are situated behind the elbows and knees, under the arms, on either side of the throat and, especially, in the groin. Skin brushing removes dead skin layers and other impurities, thereafter keeping the pores open and unclogged, and increases the elimination capacity of the skin. It is important to remember that the skin brush is exclusively yours not to be lent to or borrowed by others.

Five minutes of energetic skin brushing is equivalent to 30 minutes jogging as far as physical tone is concerned. It will build up healthy muscle tone and stimulate better distribution of fat deposits.

You will need a natural bristle brush with a detachable long wooden handle. (Nylon and synthetic fibres create static in the body and you would need to scrub for 20–30 minutes with a loofah or hand mitt to achieve the same effect as just five minutes' brushing – don't use them.) At my clinic I sell brushes made with Mexican tampico fibres which I import from Germany. The bristles are quite stiff to begin with but soften with use so start with a light pressure and increase it. Your skin should be nicely pink and glowing.

....

Do not brush on the face: a softer and smaller brush is needed for that area.

....

As your skin brushing is done dry brush on dry skin it is important to maintain the brush properly. Wash it out once a week in warm soapy water, using natural soap. Rinse it well and dry thoroughly in the airing cupboard.

How to Skin Brush

- Start with soles of your feet and a dry body. Brush upward toward the heart from below and downward from above.
- Brush vigorously up the legs and over the thighs, remembering to brush toward the groin where the lymph glands are. Use a circular clockwise movement over the abdomen, following the line of the colon, and do this about ten times.

....

Avoid the genital area and the nipples.

....

- Brush the palms and the backs of the hands, up the arms to the shoulders, then use downward strokes on the neck, throat and over the chest. To stimulate the important lymph glands under the arms you need to use your hands to create a pumping action. Lodge the thumb under the clavicle bone and with all the fingers grip the pectoral muscle making sure the fingertips get right into the armpit. Squeeze and then release this area about 15 times on each side.

- Attach the handle to the brush so that you can brush across the top of the shoulders and upper back, then up over the buttocks and lower back.
- This should take you about five minutes daily: first thing in the morning is the best time. Should you need to brush twice a day, don't brush too close to bedtime or you will not sleep. Brush every day for three months, then reduce it to two or three times weekly, changing the days each week. Never brush skin that is irritated, damaged or infected or over bad varicose veins.
- The scalp can be brushed to stimulate hair growth and to get rid of dandruff or impurities; alternatively, you may prefer to massage the scalp with your fingertips to move the scalp skin.

SHOWERING

After your five minutes' skin brushing, remove the dead skin cells by showering. Take a hot shower or bath for two to three minutes followed by a cold shower for 20 seconds and repeat seven times. Move the shower head from the feet upward and then finish by holding it over the medulla oblongata at the back of the skull, letting cold water run down the spine. This method of hydrotherapy will alkalize the blood, clean the head and give a special boost to the glandular system.

To help look after this unique and very special covering you can do several things.

- Use only natural fabrics, such as cotton, linen, silk, wool, next to the skin. That includes cotton or wool gloves and leather or canvas shoes.
- Use only natural organic soaps or olive-oil-based soaps, and natural oils which penetrate the skin rather than mineral or synthetic oils that lie on the surface only.
- Take regular exercise to promote breathing: Turkish baths and saunas also help (see page 48).
- Encourage elimination by dry skin brushing daily. When fasting skin brush twice daily, morning and evening.

THE LYMPHATIC SYSTEM

This can be best described as the body's vacuuming system. It is closely allied with the mucous membranes in the bloodstream, but unlike the blood circulation, it doesn't have a heart to act as a pump. Instead it relies on the action of the muscles and lungs to move the lymphatic fluids around the body through a one-way valve system.

The lymphatic vessels are particularly concentrated in the groin, behind the knees, in the armpits and under the chin, as well as in the top part of the chest and down the spine, but they spread like a gossamer network of tubes about the diameter of a needle throughout the body, covering every area except for the central nervous system. Lymph vessels have a vast population of white blood cells whose purpose is to attack and ingest invaders, cleaning out waste. They co-ordinate in such a way that they act as a good policing system ensuring that your auto-immune system is doing what it should. However if they falter, the lymphatic system backs up and one or more of the lymphatic nodules swells up with poisonous waste.

....

You may feel a lump or notice a bleeding or enlarged mole. At this stage your lymph system needs urgent attention. Seek the advice of a qualified medical herbalist.

....

The lymphatic system has particular difficulty in dealing with heavy metals and industrial chemicals, whether you breathe them in, put them on your skin or in your teeth or eat them.

One of the finest ways to get the lymph system moving is to trampoline (use a mini-trampoline) but don't do so if you are prone to prolapse. All muscles have got to be in pretty good shape before you start any kind of vigorous exercise so if in doubt begin with long brisk walks striding out and swinging your arms. If this is too jarring on your joints, try swimming, where you are comparatively weightless in water, but look for a pool which is free of added chlorine. There are some ozone pools around.

If the lymph is battling with heavy metals and industrial chemicals take the Intestinal Corrective Formulation No. 3 (see page 152). Couple this with Intestinal Corrective Formulation No. 2 (page 144) to assist its action. Alongside this take the following chronic purifier formula.

CHRONIC PURIFIER

Mix three parts blue flag, three parts echinacea, two parts mimosa gum, one part each comfrey root and Irish moss. This formulation is deep reaching and effective, but try to make sure your bowel is working very thoroughly before you embark on its use. Take three size 0 capsules of the finely powdered herbs three times a day.

Remember that skin brushing has a very effective action on the superficial vessels of the lymphatic system.

THE RESPIRATORY SYSTEM

Women, in general, are particularly inefficient breathers, using only the top third of their lungs. This type of laziness results in lack of vitality and an acceleration of metabolic disorders and degeneration of the tissues all over the body. Most pathological changes in such tissues can be prevented if they are constantly surrounded by life-giving oxygen. Correct breathing is the best preventative medicine of all. The problem is that most of us forget how to breathe once we get beyond the stage of nappies.

CORRECT BREATHING

You need to begin by improving your posture. Stand and sit tall and when you lie down make sure you are well stretched out. Keep your head well up and don't tuck your chin in or let it jut out. An easy way to check your posture is to stand barefoot against a wall without a skirting board, trying to flatten the whole length of your spine and the back of the head against the wall. Now stretch up and breathe out deeply. Take a step away from the wall holding this position: the way you are at this moment is how, ideally, you should stand and walk.

Avoid as far as possible polluted, including smoky, air. The correlation between low birth weight and the number of cigarettes smoked daily by mothers-to-be is now widely recognized, but not many people realize that women can affect the foetus almost as much with passive smoking. Babies are even affected by cuddling up against mothers and smelling toxins coming out of their skin.

An ionizer, which helps to control the balance of ions (tiny electrical particles) in the air around you, is particularly useful and can be plugged into the bedroom socket at night where it will do its good work while you sleep.

Mucus is normally produced as a protective barrier on the surface of membranes but when the body is irritated it is over-produced causing excessive sticky mucus in which germs are easily harboured. Mucus-forming foods include dairy products, eggs, meat, sugar, tea and coffee, chocolate, anything which is white and refined including the gluten in wheat, oats, rye and barley, potatoes, swedes, turnips and parsnips and any other starchy root vegetables. Foods which are good at cutting through mucus include nettles, kelp, onions, horseradish root, garlic and sprouted fenugreek.

SINUS TONIC

Again this is the formulation of my teacher Richard Schulze in the United States and it works superbly well. Put equal parts of finely chopped or grated fresh horseradish root, onion, ginger root, garlic and chilis into a jar and cover in cider vinegar. The easiest way to grate all this together without passing out is to put it through a food processor with a grater attachment. Macerate for two weeks from the new moon to the full moon and then strain and rebottle, stoppering tightly. Take a tablespoon before each meal.

While being made, this formulation is unbeatable for cleaning out the sinuses and makes a wonderful gargle for the throat particularly if you think you may be going down with an infection. It is very protective against invading viral and bacterial infections of the mucous membranes in the mouth, throat or upper respiratory tract. Simply gargle with it several times a day and swallow afterward.

Oil or syrup of garlic is particularly useful of treating colds, flu and chest infections as well as bronchial congestion and sore throats.

Certain essential oils used in herbal steam baths will vaporize mucus and loosen irritants. The best oil for this is fennel seed because it causes mucus to degenerate so that the eliminative process can move it through the bloodstream far more effectively than can be done by coughing, sneezing or blowing the nose. Use 10 drops of fennel oil to 1 pt (575 ml) freshly boiled water; put this in a basin and cover your head with a towel holding your face 8 in (20 cm) away from the infusion. Keeping the eyes and mouth closed breathe in and out steadily through the nose. Do this for 20 minutes at a time, repeating morning and evening.

RESPIRATORY FORMULATION

Make a decoction of three parts coltsfoot, three parts mullein, one part comfrey, one part elderflower, one part liquorice, one part lobelia and drink half a breakfast cup three times a day. This will support the respiratory system if it is actively eliminating or chronically weak.

REST

It is also important to understand that we cannot heal ourselves unless we rest. Indeed the only time cells regenerate in our body is when we are in deep meditation or fast asleep, so sleeping is vital for rejuvenation. Besides this, our dreams can carry out the nightly task of sifting through the day's unsettled problems, emotions and thoughts. Dreaming is actually therapeutic although it may make no sense to us at all. One of the simplest techniques for inducing sleep is barefoot walking on soil or grass. It discharges the excessive electrical energy built up in the body during the course of the day. Dr Christopher recounts a story in which he cured a lifetime history of insomnia in an elderly man simply by asking him to get up in the middle of the night when he was unable to sleep and put on his dressing gown. He then had to walk barefoot in his back yard for 20 minutes. Unsurprisingly the gentleman concerned was extremely sceptical but desperate enough to try it and within two weeks he was sleeping comfortably for a good six hours nightly.

To be effective barefoot walking should be carried out for a minimum of five minutes on grass, sand or soil, then the feet should be dried vigorously with a rough towel and then warm socks and dry shoes or slippers put on. (An alternative is to fill a wooden box full of builder's sand so that you can simply stand in the kitchen and walk up and down on the spot in this for five minutes.) See also page 118.

If you use any clothing at all at night, it should be natural, and sleep in cotton sheets. The bed should be well aired with some source of air coming in from the outside through a slightly open window. A healthy body will lose at least 1 pt (575 ml) of fluid overnight into the surrounding material.

There are several very simple teas that can be drunk in isolation to induce more restful sleep including the flowers of lime tree, camomile, lemon balm, hops and elder.

It is also possible to learn relaxation. The choice of methods is wide and not all methods are suitable for every person. Meditation, yoga, self-hypnosis, visualization, autogenics, bio-feedback; keep trying until you settle on a method that is right for you. Above all don't be discouraged if you are not instantly brilliant at it. After all, surely you could not learn to play a musical instrument in a week! The secret is to find a method you like and persist with it.

Regular vigorous exercise will also help you to sleep better.

CHAPTER 4

PROTECTING YOURSELF AGAINST COMMON POISONS

———

There is now no doubt that poisons in our environment cause all sorts of serious disorders, disease and death. These range from vague sub-clinical conditions like headaches, irritability, chronic mental and physical fatigue and digestive disorders to our most dreaded killers like cancer. While the chemical, drug, medical, food-processing, oil and other vested interests hold sway over the world, their main purpose is to ensure that nothing will hinder their profits. Nor can you expect the government (of any shade) to do anything about it: most governments are heavily influenced financially or politically by these interests. The only one who can help you is yourself. Imagine what would happen if you began by helping yourself and then showed your family and your relatives how to help themselves, and so on. With that spread of information, the world could be a very different place.

An American researcher, Dr H. Rudolph Alsleben, conducted an exhaustive five-year study to determine exactly what people had in their bodies. More than half a million tests on people of all ages and backgrounds were carried out. Dr Alsleben found four kinds of tissue destruction in every single person studied: these were heavy metal poisoning (lead, mercury, arsenic, cadmium, nickel and strontium), atherosclerosis, infection and malnutrition.

The good news is the damage to the body by certain common poisons in air, water and food can be minimized and even prevented by the regular use of specific foods. For example, certain foods can help the development and growth of beneficial bacteria in the intestines which in turn help to detoxify and neutralize certain toxic residues in food. A diet high in specific nutritive substances can increase the body's tolerance and resistance to toxins. Other foods can actively eliminate ingested poisons from the system.

CARBON MONOXIDE

Carbon monoxide – a chief component of exhaust gases – interferes with the oxygenation of all the cells of your body by preventing oxygen from being absorbed by your lungs. It can cause respiratory disorders, irritability, loss of memory, headaches, breathlessness, angina, emphysema, anaemia, heart disease and cancer. Vitamin E increases tissue oxygenation and decreases the body's need for oxygen by preventing the undesirable oxidation of liquids in the bloodstream. It is richly present in whole grains, nuts and their oils.

The B vitamins markedly increase the body's tolerance to oxygen deficiency caused by carbon monoxide and are richly present in nutritional yeast and whole grains. Vitamin A has a specific protective property against carbon monoxide and other toxins in polluted air; it works by increasing the permeability of blood capillaries, thereby facilitating better delivery of oxygen to the cells. It is richly present in freshly squeezed carrot juice.

There are now cars on the market which filter the air before it comes into the vehicle; if you drive in severely polluted cities, it may well be worth investing in one.

OZONE AND NITROGEN DIOXIDE

These photochemical air pollutants are the health-damaging constituents of smog. They can exacerbate respiratory disorders, notably emphysema. Vitamin A protects the mucous membranes against pollutants and vitamin E keeps the ozone from destroying vitamin A in the body.

LEAD

Lead is a neuro-toxin and can damage the brain and nervous system, causing anaemia and affecting the muscles. High levels of lead in water have been demonstrated to depress the intelligence of children. In 1987 the Medical Research Council concluded from a study commissioned in Edinburgh that most city children probably had lead levels in their bodies high enough to impede their intellectual growth and that there was no evidence of a safe level. Lead absorbed from water running through lead pipes was frequently the main source of the poison.

Studies by the Greater Glasgow Health Board in 1980 showed that mothers with a higher than average level of lead in their bloodstream suffered more stillbirths and that surviving babies tended to be born very small. Lead crosses the placenta easily. In 1980, the Government decided against removing all lead piping from British homes (as has long since been done in America) when the cost was estimated at £2bn. In the meantime the Government suggests flushing lead pipes every morning, but for this precaution to be effective, it must be done every time a tap has been turned off for 15 consecutive minutes. Few people do this and now that water usage is being metered, even fewer are likely to do so.

Lead poisoning from tap water is still widespread in schools and hospitals. In 1983 a senior water scientist found lead levels of 5,000 micrograms per litre in the children's ward of a hospital.

Other types of piping – iron, plastic, copper, lead, zinc and cement – may also leach dangerous trace elements like lead or cadmium.

The early symptoms of lead poisoning are generally vague and therefore somewhat difficult to detect. They include lack of appetite, fatigue and nervousness. As the poison accumulates in the system it will damage the kidneys, liver, heart and nervous system so that eventually, in extreme cases, there will be paralysis of the extremities, blindness, mental disturbances, mental retardation and even insanity. Chronic lead poisoning can cause sexual impotence in men.

Protection against lead includes calcium which has both a preventative and curative effect on lead poisoning by helping the body to safely excrete lead from the system. It is richly present in nuts and seeds, home-made nut milks and carrot juice. Vitamin D, richly present in natural sunlight, protects against lead poisoning, as does vitamin C, which is a powerful antitoxin, protecting muscle tissue from lead. It is richly present in dark green leafy vegetables and fruit. Vitamin B_1 is of specific value in protecting against the damaging effects of lead and is richly present in nutritional yeast. Vitamin A helps activate enzymes which are involved in detoxifying lead poisons. Lecithin is a neutralizer of poisons in the body, working specifically with the liver, and it protects the myelin sheaths of nerve fibres from being damaged by lead. Lecithin is available in health-food shops in granule or capsule form (see Resources Directory). Pulses and beans help to excrete lead from the system, as does seaweed (see Superfoods, page 18). Above all avoid smoking: smoking cigarettes can increase your daily intake of lead by up to 25%.

MERCURY

Mercury is one of the most commonly present poisons in our environment, having contaminated our soil, water and food supply. Poisoning from mercury results in brain damage, nerve paralysis and serious damage to the nervous system. It also interferes with enzyme activity, damages the kidneys and liver and causes paralysis and blindness. Protection against mercury includes nutritional yeast and garlic, which contain selenium and act as an antidote to help to destroy the mercury in the body. Calcium helps to neutralize mercury and facilitates excretion. To encourage sufficient hydrochloric acid in the stomach see the formulation on page 111 for digestive herbs. Lecithin minimizes the toxic effect of mercury.

DENTAL AMALGAMS

Despite 12,000 published papers on the dangers of amalgams, so far they have failed to alter the opinion of the majority of the dental profession in this country as to their toxicity. However, in Sweden, because mercury fillings in pregnant women are acknowledged to affect the foetus, pregnant women are no longer allowed to have such fillings. On 14–17 June 1989 the University of Calgary Medical School presented the Canadian Federation of Biological Societies with a paper that showed that amalgam fillings placed in the molar teeth of five pregnant sheep produced mercury in foetal blood and amniotic fluid within three days of being inserted. After 16 more days, the mercury was evident in the pituitary glands, liver, kidney and part of the placenta and by 33 days (which is round about the time of birth for a sheep) nearly all foetal tissue had higher levels of mercury than the tissues of the mother. During lactation the mothers had eight times as much mercury in the milk as in their own blood serum. But in the UK women are actively encouraged to have dental work during their pregnancy.

By no means does everyone react badly to mercury fillings, so you should be properly tested by someone qualified and experienced in this field (see Resources Directory). It is also vital to get the fillings removed in the right sequence by a dentist who is both experienced and fully qualified to do so. Any dentist simply won't do. Both Levenson and Higgins, respectively the British and American leaders in this field, insist that the most negatively charged fillings be taken out first. Those who find they are mercury toxic and rush off to their dentists to have their amalgam fillings replaced willy-nilly often get sicker if this protocol is not observed, because they suffer from an onslaught of mercury vapours.

If you are diagnosed as being highly sensitive to mercury (and tests done in advance can ascertain this) you should take 6 g of vitamin C mixed into water at the first signs of any adverse reactions.

DDT

It is commonly thought that the Government in the USA have banned DDT but they have, in fact, only limited it; DDT is still present everywhere throughout the world. It has been found in the breast milk of mothers in the Gobi Desert, as well as in the livers of penguins in Antartica. Because it decomposes very slowly it would take 20 or 30 years to get it out of the environment, even supposing other countries weren't using it.

DDT is a cumulative poison stored mainly in the fat tissues of the body, which means it can be found in greater amounts than elsewhere in milk and other dairy products, meat and human breast milk. Water releases DDT into the system extremely quickly which is one of the reasons I don't encourage people to fast on water alone. (I recommend always fasting on juices and potassium broth which minimizes the danger of DDT poisoning.) Lecithin binds up DDT minimizing its harmful effects and vitamin C helps to neutralize it.

CADMIUM

This is found in certain petrol, in smoggy air, in phosphate fertilizers and in our soft water supplies. Both the galvanized and newer black plastic pipes contain cadmium which is dissolved and leached out by acids in the water, particularly first thing in the morning when it has been standing in the pipes all night.

....

Hot water leaches even more than cold water and should therefore never be used for cooking or drinking.

....

Shellfish and animal livers often contain dangerous amounts of cadmium.

Cadmium poisoning can be caused by the use of enamelled utensils and pots because it is used to achieve those beautiful colours. It is dissolved by acids in food and ends up in our bodies. I work in the Potteries and have treated several painters in the industry for severe cadmium poisoning. It is even more dangerous than lead, causing high blood pressure, heart disease, iron deficiency, atherosclerosis, emphysema, chronic bronchitis, lung fibrosis, kidney damage and cancer.

Vitamin C is a specific protector against cadmium. Avoid white flour; 78% of the zinc it contains is removed from it once the bran and wheatgerm are taken out in the milling process and zinc-rich foods prevent the assimilation of cadmium. Zinc is richly present in all seeds, nuts and whole grains but particularly pumpkin and sunflower seeds. Don't use coloured enamelled utensils and drink pure filtered water.

STRONTIUM-90

There have now been so many nuclear tests worldwide that scientists acknowledge that everybody has dangerous amounts of radioactive strontium-90 in the bones and that it stays in the body throughout life, emitting radioactive rays like X-rays. Anaemia, leukaemia and bone cancer are all attributed to strontium-90 (although this is not the only cause, by any means).

Seaweed, specifically kelp, is very helpful for removing strontium-90 from the body and pectin binds it in the intestines reducing its absorption and deposition in the skeleton. The pectin found in raw sunflower seeds was found to be particularly effective for this purpose (see also Intestinal Corrective No. 3, page 152). Heavy intakes of natural calcium will reduce strontium-90 absorption by 50%. Calcium is richly present in wholegrain seeds and carrot juice. Nutritional yeast offers some protection against radiation as do lecithin and vitamins E and C.

IODINE-131

This is the result of a fallout and is believed to be even more toxic than strontium-90. It is found particularly in milk (another good reason not to let your child drink it).

It concentrates particularly in the thyroid gland (as all the children of Chernobyl discovered after the explosion) and causes thyroid cancer. Kelp is a specific protection against radioactive iodine. Follow also the protective measures for strontium-90.

X-RAYS

These have been used somewhat indiscriminately by doctors, dentists and chiropractors, as well as radiographers and hospitals. It is common knowledge that X-rays are carcinogenic, but X-rays given to 25% of all pregnant women during the 1950s and 60s may have caused between 5% and 10% of all childhood cancers throughout America and the Western world. X-rays also cause major birth defects including small head size, mental retardation, skeletal deformities and eye and heart defects. In his excellent book, *Male Practice*, Dr Robert Mendelsohn believes that the evidence is overwhelming that women who have accumulated a lot of radiation during their lives have a highly increased risk of delivering a baby with Down's syndrome and that it is this, rather than age alone, that is responsible for an older woman's increased risk. In addition, cancer research in America indicates that a specific percentage of women have inherited a gene, oncogene AC, that is sensitive to X-ray exposure and that in these particular women even very brief periods of X-ray exposure can lead to the development of cancer.

X-rays are cumulative, so even a tiny amount such as those emitted from a colour TV, a wristwatch or an alarm clock can be dangerous and add up the total amount received from all sources.

Protection includes rutin, which is richly present in buckwheat, because it strengthens the capillary walls and reduces the haemorrhaging caused by X-rays; vitamin C increases the efficacy of rutin; nutritional yeast for its B vitamins; essential fatty acids present in avocado, olive oil, flax seed, evening primrose and borage oil; the bioflavonoids present in the white pith of citrus fruits; and lecithin. The sodium alginate found in all seaweeds acts as a chelating agent, protecting the body from the harmful effects of radiation by binding them with radioactive elements and so enabling them to be excreted speedily from the body. Chaparral is a well-known protective against radiation. Chlorophyll also increases resistance to X-rays.

DRUGS

Iatrogenic illness, usually the result of surgical complications or wrongly prescribed drugs, is estimated to account for as many as 20% of all hospital admissions (up to one million annually in the USA). A British study of 750 randomly chosen coronary patients who were in similar stages of illness found that the death rate for those who were treated in intensive-care units in hospital was significantly higher than for those who were convalescing at home. And from Israel comes the interesting story that when doctors went on strike for a month in 1973, the death rate in the country dropped by 50%! In Bogotá, premature babies strapped on to the chest of their mothers did far better than those reared in intensive-care units.

Our general health is deteriorating while we are surrounded by an abundance of food, more leisure, increased education and all the other factors which, it was once assumed, would lead to greater general well-being. The majority of people in the Western world take daily medication of some sort (including synthetic vitamins and other supplements), approximately half of which has been prescribed by a doctor and the other half not.

Anything taken into the body changes its chemistry and any substance powerful enough to have an effect is capable of harm as well as good. Most of us use nicotine, alcohol and caffeine on a regular basis which means that we are permanently under the influence of something. In *Medical Nemesis* Ivan Illich argues that the increasing medicalization of modern life not only produces clinical iatrogenic illness, but obscures the effect of the social conditions which are making us unhealthy, as well as eroding our belief in our ability to heal ourselves. 'Modern medicine has become a major threat to health and its potential for social, even physical, disruption is rivalled by the perils inherent in the industrialized production of food.'

His questioning of our belief in medical solutions was echoed by the well-known immunologist, Sir Frank Macfarlane Burnet. 'The real problem of today is to find some means of diminishing the incidence of diseases of civilization. Nothing from the laboratory seems to have any relevance in such matters.'

Infectious diseases, contrary to public understanding, are not a thing of the past. Widespread and rapid international travel has made the transmission of these, as well as virulent influenza and AIDS, virtually uncontrollable.

The modern picture of illness in our society shows that the largest area consists of chronic states such as circulatory disorders, obesity, arthritis, alcoholism and other addictions and psychiatric illness. Although some of the symptoms of these illnesses can be alleviated, they are difficult to cure. The second largest group of disorders includes upper respiratory tract infections, allergies and stress-related conditions such as tension headaches, anxiety states and ulcers. These are generally treated by medication, either prescribed by a doctor or self-administered.

The medical or surgical conditions in which technical intervention is of benefit – and the ones to which the majority of medical education and public health spending is devoted – form the smallest group of all. Medicine, at the interface of humanity and technology, is still putting its energy for the most part into the technology, while the instance of illness which cannot be treated in this way is burgeoning.

Eli Lilley, the founder of one of the biggest drug companies in the world, said, 'No drug is worth its name without side effects'. Drugs destroy vital nutrition in the body and prevent its absorption, as well as damaging the liver and kidneys and causing serious diseases.

The two most commonly prescribed families of drugs are the antibiotics and sedative hypnotics, including tranquillizers and sleeping pills. Although the antibiotics are one of the most specifically successful drugs in treating bacterial infections, their overuse has led to many strains of bacteria now being resistant to them. They are sometimes prescribed for viral illnesses like flu on which they can have no effect, and many people are also getting substantial additional doses in the meat and dairy products they eat.

The second group of drugs is often prescribed to deal with a range of symptoms which really require changes in lifestyle, such as learning how to relax, how to handle stress and how to make better decisions that lead to peace of mind.

Sedative hypnotics are by no means harmless. So-called minor tranquillizer addiction is now a major problem, especially among women. These drugs are even more dangerous when taken in combination with alcohol (which is often the case). Dependence occurs if these drugs are used for any length of time, and withdrawal from them is a dangerous and difficult process. In 1984, 6.5 million prescriptions for these drugs were issued in Australia. For a country with a population of 16 million that seems an indication of something seriously wrong.

A full stomach slows down the absorption of most drugs and some are actually weaker when taken with food because they become stuck to food components. For example, digoxin given for heart disease can become attached to bran and tetracyclines become bonded to milk. The way drugs are removed from the body is by the long-suffering liver and kidneys; drugs which specifically damage the liver include paracetamol, sulphonamides (which are used to treat infections), salicylates (used to relieve pain and inflammation), rifampicin (for treating TB), antibiotics, chemotherapy drugs (used for cancer), certain types of anaesthetics, phenothiazines (for treating psychosis and schizophrenia) and many steroids including oral contraceptives and drugs used for diabetes and thyroid problems.

For liver protection and detoxification see page 80. Cysteine, one of the natural amino acids, acts as an antioxidant in the liver, as does selenium which is richly present in garlic, onions, comfrey, radish and horseradish.

If anything, the kidneys are even more sensitive than the liver to drug damage. Almost every drug can affect the kidneys, sometimes irreversibly. To protect the kidneys the diet needs to be alkaline: alkaline foods include fruits, vegetables, nuts, grains and seeds. Of all these, the most alkaline is potassium broth (see page 31). Kidneys also appreciate a low-protein diet, so this is yet another good reason for eating a vegan diet.

Some drugs are eliminated by bile from the liver. A diet with plenty of roughage and good bacteria in the intestines helps its production, as does the liver flush on page 81. Remember, garlic produces good intestinal flora as does bioacidophilus (for suppliers see Resources Directory). If you have to take any kind of drug (except penicillin and antibiotics) take large doses of vitamin C. The acid in vitamin C breaks up the penicillin and antibiotics prematurely. Also take lots of lecithin, vitamin B complex and vitamin E. Avoid all alcohol, refined oils, animal fats, salt, additives and preservatives, chemicals of any kind, smoking and meat and dairy products.

PESTICIDES

Healthy soil is one of the world's greatest natural resources, yet this rich nutrient-packed layer of the earth's crust from which food crops draw their sustenance is currently being lost at the rate of 24 billion tonnes a year. This is the result of intensive farming with large amounts of chemical fertilizers, coupled with monoculture and the ploughing up of margin lands. What is at stake here is not only the degradation of soil but the degradation of life itself.

One billion gallons of liquid pesticide are now being used yearly on Britain's farms. The London Food Commission conducted a thorough toxicological survey on the active ingredients permitted to be used by UK pesticide manufacturers currently. Nearly 40% of these pesticides were linked with at least one adverse effect. Of the 426 chemicals listed, 68 were carcinogenic, 61 capable of mutating genes, 35 had various reproductive effects ranging from impotence to a variety of birth defects, and 93 caused skin irritations and other somewhat milder complications. The biggest culprits were herbicides, especially the carboxyacid and phenylurea groups, as well as chlorinated desolvents.

It has long been proven that there is a higher incidence of cancers and related disorders in those people occupationally exposed to pesticides. The disorders include cancer of the lung, kidney and testicles, leukaemia and multiple types of tumours, non-Hodgkin's lymphomas and malignant lymphomas, brain tumours and soft-tissue sarcomas. Pesticides can also cause damage to the genetic material of young children (witness the spina bifida and facial clefts of those children born to US servicemen exposed during the Vietnam War to Agent Orange). Pesticides have a toxic effect on the brain of children causing measurable changes in brain function as well as aggression, memory difficulties, depression, schizophrenic reactions and other emotional instability. Besides this they cause active brain degeneration including some of the sclerosing diseases like multiple sclerosis, muscular dystrophy and Guillain Barré-like syndromes.

Chronic exposure to pesticides disrupts the way our immune systems work, resulting in allergies and other immuno-regulatory disorders including chronic fatigue syndrome and myalgic encephalomyelitis.

The use of nitrogen fertilizers affects the nutritional value of crops. This can cause alarmingly low levels of manganese, zinc and iron. It has now been proven that organic food contains a much higher level of nutrients than inorganic food. The US National Academy of Sciences monitored 14 successful organic farms over five years and found some had corn yields that were 32% higher and soya bean yields that were 40% higher than local farms using pesticides.

The problem is that most of what we eat is subject to high and frequently repeated doses of chemicals. Cereal crops like wheat get sprayed five to eight times during a growing season and some vegetables and fruit crops 10 to 15 times. Once harvested, they are sprayed again to protect them from storage disease. Pesticides are used in sheep dips, warble-fly dressings, lice treatment, and in veterinary pesticides for controlling flies and other insects in livestock.

Local authorities use huge amounts of pesticides in their parks, lawns, gardens, golf courses and other recreational grounds, and railway contractors spray thousands of pounds of pesticides into railway embankments. Those who maintain the canals and various waterways use large quantities of pesticides to remove excessive weeds.

Electrical cables are doused with insecticide and lindane is used by modern builders to preserve wood. Pesticides are also ubiquitous in wallpaper pastes, wooden furniture, do-it-yourself products and natural-fibre textiles. They are present in many baby foods, and have been found in drinking water in the UK with nearly a quarter of samples taken exceeding the maximum admissible concentration. Besides industrial pollutants and pesticides, nitrates are also widely present in drinking water as the result of the burgeoning use of nitrogen-based fertilizers spread on to the soil. It is estimated that approximately one million people in the UK are exposed to nitrate levels in drinking water that exceed the present maximum admissible concentration, and that this will quadruple by the turn of the century.

AVOIDING PESTICIDES

Aim to eat as much organic food as possible and if you are eating meat and dairy produce ensure that this too is organic. If you can't find organic foods, write to organizations that might be able to help you (see Resources Directory). In the meantime, buy fruits and vegetables from reputable supermarket chains because they generally have fairly strict monitoring and quality control and therefore their shelves will be full of foods with lower levels of pesticide residues. At the same time, demand organic foods in every shop and supermarket you enter. If enough people shout loudly you can be sure retailers will listen.

Wash all fruits and vegetables, especially leafy vegetables, and fruits with skin that can be eaten. (However, washing removes only a small amount of pesticides so peeling is safer.) Even then, peeling won't remove all the residues because some find their way into the flesh. Always use filtered water to drink and to cook with. Use organic pesticides in your own garden or learn about the protection that planting herbs among fruits, vegetables and decorative plants can afford your garden. Use organic pesticides only when you are certain that they are absolutely necessary and use them sparingly. Store all pesticides away from food, children and pets, well locked up.

Take the trouble to write to your MP demanding better pesticide safety control. At the moment levels of pesticides in our food and water are very poorly controlled. For example, a survey conducted by the Association of Public Analysts in 1983 found a third of all fruits and vegetables sampled to be contaminated with pesticide residues. There are washes designed to remove pesticides (see Resources Directory).

NITRATES AND NITRITES

Processed meats are preserved with these and even innocuous baby foods contain nitrates. Nitrates and nitrites are converted into nitrosamines in the intestine. Nitrosamines are carcinogenic, causing cancer in the liver, stomach, brain, oesophagus, bladder, kidneys and several other organs. They also cause high blood pressure and heart disease, and interfere with the conversion of carotene into vitamin A in the body.

In acute cases of poisoning large doses of vitamin C help, preventing the conversion of nitrates and nitrites into nitrosamines. Besides these the vitamin B complex contained in nutritional yeast as well as vitamins A and E and lecithin have been found to be effective in neutralizing their damaging effects.

GENERAL PROTECTIVE MEASURES

In general, it is not the isolated poisons but the continual accumulative toxic assault that matters.

We are victims of the boiling frog principle. If a frog is put into hot water it will do everything it can to escape it. It knows beyond a shadow of a doubt it can't survive such an extreme environment. But if it is put into cold water that is heated up slowly, it doesn't struggle, it adapts bit by bit, until it is dead. We adapt to the chemical contamination of our environment little by little, as the toxic residue in our tissues increases. However chemicals not normally found in the body are unsafe at any dosage. There is no safe level. In spite of this, we are exposed to them constantly, every time we sit in a car or in a plastic chair or in a painted room.

If you have a choice move out of the city or get out into the countryside as often as you can. Make sure you breathe clean air for at least the few weeks a year you have on holiday. Make every effort to eat only organically grown foods or grow your own. Anyone can sprout their own seeds. There are various washes that you can buy on the market (see Resources Directory) to wash chemicals off the skins of fruit and vegetables and those fruits and vegetables that cannot be washed should be peeled. Obviously, stop adding to the problem and be part of the solution by not using any more toxic chemicals in your house or garden. If you have to dry clean your clothes, ventilate them for several days after the cleaning. Above all ensure that you get the best possible diet into you and your family.

CHAPTER 5

THE HOLISTIC FAMILY MEDICAL HERBAL

———

Note: Many of these illnesses can be diagnosed through iridology. Iridology is the study of the neuro-optic reflex. To the trained and experienced practitioner, the iris of the eye reveals inherent characteristics of body tissue, the presence of toxic metals, acids, catarrh and anaemia, through which it is possible to gauge the acute, chronic and destructive stage of any organ. The relationships of various organs to the autonomic and nervous systems can be determined, as well as whether the endocrine glands are hyper- or hypo-active (over- or under-active). Iridology can also act as preventative tool by revealing a predisposition to certain disorders and disease processes long before they have reached the awareness threshold. It is, therefore, a wonderful tool for assessing a person holistically.

ABSCESSES AND BOILS

An abscess is a localized collection of pus, known as a whitlow on the finger, as a gum boil on the jaw, and as a boil on any part of the skin. It is possible to develop abscesses internally in the breast, kidney and brain, and internal infections need professional treatment. Most of us have experienced a boil at some time or another as the result of local irritation by a hair follicle or a splinter. Repeated boils and abscesses, however, are generally the result of auto-intoxication, or toxaemia, that is, the body is overloaded with poisons. Very occasionally diabetes or an allergy may cause boils. Wherever abscesses and boils are chronic, embark on deep internal cleansing (see juice fasting, page 29), paying special attention to the glandular system, blood, liver and bowels.

Ice placed locally on a boil in its early stages will often abort its development but for chronic boils it is better to encourage deep internal cleansing. Do not attempt to lance boils as infection can easily be spread.

POULTICE

My favourite poultice for boils is a flax seed one. Grind equal parts of organic flax seeds and peeled garlic in a liquidizer and boil both together to a porridge-like *consistency with filtered water. Start with 1 oz (30 g) each, and adjust quantities according to the size of the boil or abscess. Renew the poultice twice daily, first showering off using the hot/cold shower routine (page 50).*

Tea-tree oil applied six times a day is also helpful and organic honey poured straight into deep ulcerated sores is excellent for chronic abscesses. Besides supporting the body's channels of elimination (bowels, skin, lungs, liver, lymph system and kidneys), take two herbal antibiotics every half hour while awake.

ACNE

This is characterized by various skin changes ranging from blackheads through to pustules and papules which are usually found on the face, although sometimes they extend to the shoulders, back, arms and chest. Their cause is hormonal and dietary which is why acne affects 80% of all teenagers to some extent. Infantile acne just after birth is the result of high levels of circulating sex hormones. Before the middle of this century the Canadian Inuits had no incidence of acne but as more modern foods, including sugar and refined carbohydrates, were introduced acne became common among them.

DIET

A wholefood vegan diet is advisable because saturated fats aggravate the problem. Cold-pressed unsaturated vegetable oils are permissible in small quantities but they should not be heated, which means that no food should be served fried. In some people iodine aggravates acne so it is as well to avoid kelp as well as iodized table salt in the diet. Deficiencies including zinc, vitamins A and B complex as well as selenium aggravate the condition and since acne is always worsened by emotional stress and imbalance, total relaxation and peace of mind are essential prerequisites for healing.

EXTERNAL TREATMENTS

Use mild natural soaps (see Resources Directory) for cleansing both the skin and the hair and expose the face to sun and fresh air as often as possible. Poultices of grated cucumber, cooked puréed organic carrots or pinhead oatmeal cooked in water are helpful. Leave the poultice on as a face mask for half an hour and then wash off with cold water. Cleanse the skin regularly with equal parts of lemon juice and purified water. At night before going to bed massage equal parts of sesame, sunflower, flax seed, almond and olive oil sparingly but thoroughly into the skin. This formulation will feed the skin, helping it to revitalize and restoring its normal activity. To bring out lesions steam the face over hot water mixed with ten drops of tea-tree oil and then dab the spots with marigold tincture or a cube of ice after the treatment. Avoid hot baths and showers and instead take alternating hot and cold showers using a mild soap (see page 50).

HERBS

On rising do a liver flush every morning (see page 80). Herbs which help to drain the lymphatic system and cleanse the liver and the bloodstream, as well as the bowel, are called for. The following tea should be drunk three times a day and dosage adjusted according to age.

Two parts of:
echinacea
burdock
dandelion
Oregon grape root
yellow dock
red clover
Prepare as a decoction and drink unsweetened.

Remember that it takes between 20 and 30 days for the skin to be formed internally before it reaches the surface; as a result persistence is necessary for true healing.

ALCOHOLISM

Liver disease, high blood pressure, irritability, tremors, slurred speech, inability to think, depression and fatigue are the long-term effects of too much alcohol, which also has an adverse affect upon the body's metabolism and its nutritional state. A pint of beer contains 250 calories, with the result that obesity can also be a problem, as can damage to the oesophagus, stomach and pancreas, an increased risk of gout and elevated cholesterol levels. Alcoholism can also exacerbate diabetes and heart disease, damage the brain and nervous system and increase the risk of developing cancer of the liver, oesophagus, larynx and mouth. Women who drink during pregnancy risk giving birth to a child with foetal alcohol syndrome, characterized by facial deformities or mental retardation.

Malnutrition usually precedes alcoholism and is aggravated by it, and 95% of all alcoholics are hypoglycaemic (alcohol gives a faster sugar boost than sucrose). The commonly held view that alcoholics are psychologically sick or simply lazy and irresponsible is generally inaccurate. In my experience, alcoholic addiction is rare in people following a good diet. In one experiment, one group of rats was fed on unrefined carbohydrates and supplemental vitamins, another on the refined carbohydrate diet typical of most hypoglycaemics and a third group on unrefined carbohydrates and high protein, a diet successfully used to treat hypoglycaemia. Each group was supplied with water and alcohol (not mixed). The group fed refined carbohydrate, which is known to exacerbate hypoglycaemia, began to prefer alcohol over water almost entirely while the low-protein group drank a little alcohol and the group fed unrefined carbohydrates and high protein avoided the alcohol altogether. This study demonstrates that if hypoglycaemia is allowed to develop, ideal conditions exist for the development of alcoholism.

TREATMENT

Begin with a two-week vegetable juice fast to normalize blood sugar and stop the physiological alcoholic addiction. Ensure at least six to eight heaped teaspoons of spirulina are added to the juice throughout the day. In my experience in treating alcoholics there is usually no craving for alcohol during this period of fasting, which gives a flying to start toward breaking the drinking habit, so helping to remove not only the physical dependence but the psychological factors.

The diet should then be a hypoglycaemic diet of high fibre with adequate protein divided into six small meals daily; fruit juices are banned although fresh fruit may be eaten. Home-made nut milks and Fruit Smoothies (as these contain frozen fruit which slows digestion) with plenty of Superfood added are very helpful (see page 31).

DELIRIUM TREMENS

This results from coming off a high intake of alcohol abruptly. Withdrawal symptoms include mental confusion, memory loss, hallucinations, shaking, sweating, agitation, insomnia, a fast pulse and high blood pressure, which may go on for several days. Such symptoms can be eased with equal parts of skullcap and lady's slipper brewed as a decoction and sweetened with organic maple syrup. Drink a quarter of a cup hot every hour until the DTs subside.

Delirium tremens requires immediate professional medical treatment.

OTHER AIDS

Angelica tea is known to create a distaste for alcohol. Evening primrose oil, 4,000 mg daily, softens the affected alcohol withdrawal and if liver function is impaired take a liver flush every morning, adding 60 drops of the liver herbs to it (see page 80).

Check that herbal and allopathic medications do not contain alcohol because even a teaspoon of alcohol will restimulate cravings. Most herbal preparations contain less than this; if in doubt, put a herbal tincture into freshly boiled water and allow the water to cool in order to evaporate the alcohol. Alcoholics Anonymous is a very useful programme to help break the psychological addiction to alcohol and establish positive associations with liquid intake. (See Resources Directory.)

ALLERGIES

Over the last decade allergies have proliferated. Is it any wonder when you consider the plethora of chemically processed foods and other irritants our overburdened livers have to neutralize? The problem is that most allergy specialists have no holistic tools with which to diagnose the cause of the problem, and treat only its symptoms. This is where iridology comes into its own.

Accurate diagnosis is obviously vital for the treatment of every illness but this is especially the case with allergies. An allergy may be the result of:

- adrenal exhaustion
- improper weaning
- specific food intolerance
- enzyme deficiency
- poor elimination
- a permeable bowel
- chemicals
- heavy metal poisoning
- chlorinated or fluoridated water
- drugs
- radiation
- sensitivity to inhaled substances
- spinal lesions
- immune system disturbance
- intestinal infection
- liver disorders
- it may be psychosomatic.

I have encountered patients who have put themselves, or worse still their children, on severe elimination diets, often on their doctor's advice, only to find they are not suffering from a food allergy at all, and in following the special diet they have become malnourished. This is particularly worrying in the case of children, who need all the necessary nutrients all the time to continue to grow and develop normally. Others have struggled with symptoms like migraines, mouth ulcers, fluid retention, depression and even in one case schizophrenia without realizing the root cause was an allergy.

FASTING

Fast for five days on vegetable juice made from organically grown vegetables only. Carrot juice makes a good, bland base to which to add smaller quantities of other vegetable juices. A teaspoon of horseradish or garlic juice is particularly helpful if the nose and eyes are streaming. Add this to 8 fl oz (250 ml) of carrot juice. Aim to drink 1 fl oz (30 ml) of carrot juice daily for every 1 lb/450 g of body weight.

If poor production of digestive enzymes is the problem add 5 fl oz (150 ml) of pineapple juice to 10 fl oz (300 ml) of pawpaw juice and 1 teaspoon of sprouted alfalfa juice.

For general strengthening of the system take 8 fl oz (250 ml) of carrots, 4 fl oz (100 ml) of celery and 4 fl oz (100 ml) of beetroot, with 1 fl oz (30 ml) of fresh parsley juice.

Generally, it is better not to fast on fruit juices since they tend to aggravate the symptoms in a significant number of patients. I disapprove of water fasting for similar reasons. A water fast alters thyroid hormone function and increases the production of hormones like cortisol from the adrenal cortex, making the patient temporarily and artificially well to such an extent that every food which is consequently reintroduced causes a violent reaction.

After the fifth day, take one food back at a time beginning with other vegetables including sprouted seeds, then fruit, then nuts and grains. Leave any food containing colouring or preservatives until last. They are the main offenders. Gradually reintroduce alcohol, chicken and hen's eggs, chocolate, tea and coffee, citrus fruits, anything that comes from a cow, including its flesh, peanuts, pork, sugar of any colour, wheat, oats, rye and corn, yeast. When introducing grains test each one for two consecutive days as they can cause a delayed reaction. It is advisable to stay on an imaginative 80% raw food diet consisting of fruit, vegetables, nuts, sprouted grains and seeds for 12 weeks. If you cannot do this at least eliminate any food that causes a reaction until you have been through your healing process. It may then be possible to introduce small quantities of the culprit food sporadically once the whole body is stronger.

....

Don't put children on a fast – get professional help.

....

HERBS FOR ALLERGY

Equal parts of:
barberry root
borage
cayenne
dandelion root
ginger
ginseng (preferably Siberian)
hawthorn berries
liquorice.
Take one level teaspoon of the finely powdered herb mixture in vegetable juice three times daily. If you have high blood pressure avoid the liquorice and substitute motherwort instead. A minimum course of three months is recommended. If further treatment is necessary seek the advice of a consultant medical herbalist.

GENERAL AIDS

Stop smoking, and consider coming off the contraceptive pill, which is a major cause of stress. The hormones in the pill can have side effects, including increased risk of cervical cancer, thrombosis, raised blood pressure, diabetes, migraines, oedema, fluid retention and weight gain, thrush and depression, and affect nutrition. They increase the need for vitamins C, B_6, B_2, B_{12} and folic acid, E, K and zinc and affect the proper metabolism of B_1. They can also exacerbate food allergies.

Eat only natural unprocessed foods and try to ensure your meat is organically raised, avoid allopathic drugs if you can, limit alcohol to moderate quantities with meals only. If you are asthmatic avoid wine, which may contain metabisulphite and will contain yeast, both of which can trigger a reaction. Organic wine is available by mail order and from larger supermarkets but, as with all wine, it is fermented and will obviously contain yeast, so even this is best avoided if a yeast allergy is suspected. It does not contain metabisulphite.

Ionizers sometimes prove helpful to people sensitive to inhalant allergens. Get plenty of sleep, sunlight and clean air and above all exercise; this will produce endorphins and encephalins which heighten the sense of well-being and stimulate the metabolism.

ALOPECIA SEE BALDNESS

ANAEMIA

Most of the time iron deficiency goes totally unrecognized; this is worrying because it is the most common worldwide nutritional disease. Symptoms include listlessness, fatigue, a very obvious heart beat on exertion, a sore tongue, cracks at the corner of the mouth, difficulty swallowing, concave nails or pale nails with vertical ridges in them, brittle, wiry, thin, lacklustre hair, loss of sexual interest, and in children poor appetite, retarded growth and an ability to catch every infection going.

Iron deficiency is the precursor of anaemia and doctors often ignore it if they can find no clear evidence of anaemia, but iron deficiency can exist without any blood changes and without the person becoming anaemic. A study in Canada showed that 19% of the population were iron deficient although only 2% were actually anaemic. Certainly, I find iron deficiency worryingly common in my own practice.

A further cause of anaemia is cellular obstruction: all the nutrients in the world are irrelevant if they never reach the cells. For this reason, many naturopaths routinely fast some anaemic patients because haemoglobin levels escalate rather than drop during a fast (any fast stimulates the blood-forming tissues to function more effectively). It is essential that the type of anaemia is established before any naturopathic treatment is begun and blood tests should include, as well as haemoglobin level and a complete blood count, serum, iron, B_{12}, folic acid, iron-bonding capacity, a serum ferritun and free erythrocyte protoporphyrin level. Iron deficiency is more common in infancy, puberty and pregnancy, during a heavy period and any other conditions causing sudden or chronic blood loss such as a chronic bleeding ulcer. Vegetarians are particularly at risk because iron absorption is impaired by whole grains, soya and other legumes although vitamin C improves the absorption of iron and most of my vegetarian patients eat a diet abundant in this vitamin. Tea and coffee taken with food radically reduce iron absorption and the stronger the brew the greater the reduction in iron absorption. People who have malabsorption problems, those living on exclusion diets for whatever reason and those producing very little gastric acid following the removal of part of the stomach, are at high risk.

The problem with synthetic iron is that it causes stomach upsets, constipation and black stools. Over-consumption of inorganic iron, a problem among the elderly who are heavily targeted by pharmaceutical companies, can lead to serious liver, pancreatic and heart problems and cause a form of arthritis. Natural sources of iron are assimilated much more easily into the body and it can help with the assimilation of vitamins C and E, as well as having the added advantage of burning up accumulated poisonous waste, flushing it out of the body. It does not cause constipation.

The richest herbal sources of iron are undoubtedly parsley and yellow dock.

....

Pregnant women should avoid very large intakes of parsley as it can stimulate smooth uterine muscle and lead to miscarriage. (Sprinkling fresh parsley on food in general is fine.)

....

All dark green leafy vegetables, especially the green tops of turnips and beets, are high in iron as is dried fruit, bananas, grapes, and beet and black cherry juice.

Women lose 15–30 mg of iron with each period and as much as 50 mg during childbirth; pregnant women need up to 120 mg a day. An excellent iron supplement is 40 drops of yellow dock tincture morning and evening in a little water or juice on an empty stomach. Do not drink tea, coffee or chocolate while taking this formula and use herbal teas and coffee substitutes instead.

If the stomach is not producing enough hydrochloric acid (its level may be determined by an iridology test) mix a teaspoon of cider vinegar in a little water half an hour before a meal and drink it. This will help the production of hydrochloric acid. It is very common for those over 40 to be deficient in hydrochloric acid and it is particularly suspect if food emerges in the stools in an almost unchanged condition, as well as in those with a problem with belching, vomiting or nausea.

ANAL FISSURE SEE HAEMORRHOIDS AND ANAL FISSURE

ANGINA SEE HEART DISEASE

ANOREXIA NERVOSA

This kills upward of 20% of its sufferers; death does not always result from the obvious starvation, but also as the result of infections and heart disorders. I found that getting an anorexic patient to accept herbs is a battle in itself but liquid zinc, which is easily swallowed in drinks and is quick to ingest, has been found to be extremely helpful, as has 0.5 mg of eagle vine (condurango) dried bark a day, and liver herbs such as gentian and barberry in tincture form.

Anorexia is extremely serious and needs urgent medical intervention as well as skilled psychological counselling – do not attempt to treat this disease at home.

ANXIETY

The link between nutrition and behaviour has been recognized for hundreds of years. Modern doctors are increasingly accepting that diet may play a role in many mental disorders including schizophrenia, manic depression, anxiety and hyperactivity. It is also well recognized that prolonged stress or severe depression results in the rapid use of many nutrients above and beyond the body's normal supply. So it is common for a stressful situation to result in nutritional deficiency even when the diet is normally adequate. During the Second World War, concentration camp prisoners, who lived on appalling diets and in very stressful conditions for a long period of time, were found to be B_3 deficient and, even after returning to a normal diet and bearable stress levels, a large percentage could only maintain mental and physical health with enormous doses of vitamin B_3. It seems that a long-term deficiency of B_3 eventually leads to a permanent excessive need for this vitamin. And, since rats reprieved of zinc have shown a dependency on extra zinc for up to three generations, psychological similarities between parents and children are not impossible.

Other causes of anxiety include:

- hypoglycaemia (any sudden drop in blood sugar levels can cause lethargy and depressive tendencies)
- diabetes and food intolerance
- reaction to food additives, preservatives and pesticides
- heavy metal toxicity including cadmium, lead and mercury
- endocrine imbalances (many women are aware of frequent emotional swings with their menstrual cycle)
- hypothyroidism, which may be a cause of lethargy and depression.

For all of these reasons before I begin to treat anxiety, depression or any other emotional disorder, I evaluate blood sugar abnormalities, food intolerances and endocrine imbalances, as well as the state of the thyroid, and I check for heavy metal toxicity. Whatever the problem I ensure that coffee, cigarettes or other tobacco, alcohol, sugar and any unnecessary drugs are entirely removed from the daily regime and that occupational sources of toxins are also eliminated.

Physical symptoms of anxiety apart from fatigue may include weakness, sweating, trembling, breathlessness, choking, fainting, hypertension, palpitations, digestive upsets, over-dependence on alcohol, drugs or tobacco, loss of interest in sex, insomnia, or simply a succession of mysterious aches, tingling, pains and niggling discomforts. Valium is the largest-selling prescription drug in the world today and women users outnumber men by a huge margin. But allopathic prescriptions merely mask the symptoms; they do nothing to deal with the social, environmental and physical conditions which are generally the cause.

It is now acknowledged that anti-anxiety drugs are addictive and it is here that herbs can play an invaluable part in helping the patient to withdraw from them. Counselling, a good diet, plenty of exercise, the support of loving friends and stress-management techniques like meditation, yoga, self-hypnosis, visualization, autogenics or bio-feedback are also necessary.

Prolonged use of any of the benzodiazepines will produce withdrawal symptoms if stopped abruptly. Doses in excess of 40 mg daily for three months will produce withdrawal symptoms, although I have observed some very sensitive patients experience withdrawal symptoms on smaller, shorter-term doses. Benzodiazepines include chlordiazepoxide, diazepam, nitrazepam, flurazepam, clorazepate, lorazepam and oxazepam, under such familiar trade names as Librium, Valium, Mogadon, Dalmane, Tranxene and Ativan. Withdrawal symptoms include anxiety, problems with breathing and, occasionally, convulsions, as well as severe emotional and perceptive change, such as seeing glittering lights, unsteadiness and experiencing noises and sensations of motion even while resting. Diazipam, Mogadon and lorazepam withdrawal can cause temporary but quite severe insomnia.

Weaning long-term users off Ativan, Serenid and Euhypnos, which are stronger, is harder than getting people off Librium, Valium, Mogadon, Dalmane and Tranxene but it is here that herbal remedies act as a useful bridge as the dosages of the chemical medicines are slowly and gently reduced. Herbs will actively tone, strengthen and nourish a nervous system which has been exposed to the heavy chemical stress of allopathic tranquillizers. Both valerian and skullcap initially replace the benzodiazepine's effects while strengthening the nervous system, easing withdrawal symptoms. After three months switch to alternative milder herbs like camomile, catnip, hops, lavender, lemon balm, lime flowers, pasque flowers, red clover, rosemary, vervain, motherwort, woodruff, oats and the ginsengs, which all have a useful part to play in supporting the body during the process of withdrawal. All of these are more easily digested in tea form.

....

Note: If you have been taking any of the allopathic tranquilizers for longer than eight weeks it is unwise to try and wean yourself off them without the support and advice of a qualified medical herbalist. Neither valerian nor skullcap should be used long term.

....

GENERAL NERVE TONIC

Equal parts of:
skullcap
valerian
lobelia
lemon balm
black cohosh
hops
ginger.
Make a tincture and take two to three teaspoons three times daily stirred into a hot drink.

APPENDICITIS

It used to be all the rage to remove even a healthy appendix if an operation on the right-hand side of the abdomen presented itself. However the appendix is a lymph aggregate and is specifically required to produce antiseptic lubricating fluid for the part of the colon where faecal matter has to travel upward against gravity with some difficulty. About the size of a small pencil, the appendix, if blocked by impacted faeces, quickly becomes inflamed and infected. Initial symptoms include colicky central abdominal pains, nausea and vomiting and, as the inflammation spreads, so the whole of the surrounding area begins to hurt badly. An acute attack may come on very suddenly and result in peritonitis, which is dangerous and needs urgent medical attention.

Grumbling appendix will often go on spasmodically for months or even years and in this case a thorough bowel cleanse is imperative.

Dr Jethro Kloss recommends a herbal enema of equal parts of spearmint, catnip, white oak bark, bayberry (or wild alum root) made as a standard decoction and administered at 2°F below body temperature. This is followed by hot and cold compresses to the appendix and the full length of the spine. At night he recommends a poultice of one part granulated or powdered lobelia to three parts crushed mullein leaves and a generous sprinkle of ginger powder. The herbs are mixed into a paste with powdered slippery elm or corn meal and a poultice is applied as warm as possible over the appendix until it has cooled. When suffering an attack of grumbling appendicitis go immediately on to a liquid fast, drinking plenty of potassium broth and fruit juice, as well as several cups of slippery elm gruel daily.

When using this combination of compresses and a decocted enema, be absolutely certain you are suffering from grumbling and not acute appendicitis. Grumbling appendix generally takes the form of recurring attacks of abdominal pain on the lower right side but the pain is dull not acute and often accompanied by a rise in temperature, nausea and sometimes vomiting.

Acute pain is very serious and needs immediate medical intervention.

In the case of grumbling appendix drink two parts echinacea, two parts wild yam, one part agrimony, one part camomile, and half a part liquorice made into a decoction. Take three cups daily for several months.

ARTHRITIS AND RHEUMATISM

As far as naturopathic treatment is concerned, it is not necessary to differentiate between the various sorts of rheumatism and arthritis. Naturopaths consider all rheumatic diseases to be induced by too much acid in the body and therefore they respond particularly well to the alkaline action of raw juices and potassium broth, both of which dissolve the accumulation of deposits around the joints and in other tissues. A mixture of equal parts of carrot, celery and beetroot juice with two tablespoons of green juice added to each 8 fl oz glass (250 ml), together with liberal quantities of potassium broth, are specifics for arthritis and other rheumatic diseases.

While the path to recovery may be long and arduous (and in my experience it undoubtedly is) recovery the natural way is absolutely possible. Certainly allopathic medicine has been used to control the pain of arthritis and rheumatism but I have never encountered anyone who has ever done anything other than get worse on conventional drugs. One of the most commonly prescribed drugs, aspirin, reduces vitamin C levels, damages connective tissue and if taken in large doses can cause the lining of the stomach to bleed. It also increases uric acid levels, depresses the adrenal glands and in large doses can lead to paralysis of the respiratory centre. Its prolonged use can cause dizziness, severe respiratory distress and mental confusion. Cortisone – the other popular drug prescribed for arthritis – depresses the adrenal glands and causes calcium depression, which in the long term results in osteoporosis.

DIET

One of the causes of rheumatism and arthritis is an accumulation of poisons or waste products in the affected tissue and a major contributing factor to this is an inappropriate diet containing foods that the body cannot tolerate or devitalized adulterated foods. Avoid all foods known to impede mineral absorption, including tea, coffee, bran and any form of flour. Plants of the Solanaceae family are known to affect some people adversely so avoid tomatoes, peppers, aubergines, tobacco and potatoes for several months and then re-introduce them and see if your condition gets worse. Heavy meat consumption is a contributing factor to arthritis because meat contains anything from 20 to 50 times more phosphorus than calcium. This stimulates the parathyroid gland which is responsible for the mobilization of calcium from the bones. The extra calcium is consequently deposited around the joints, which explains the less dense bones and calcium build-up around the articulations of an arthritic. A good vegetarian or – better still – vegan diet has a better phosphorus–calcium ratio (vegetarians tend to suffer less from arthritis than meat eaters).

FASTING

Repeated vegetable juice fasts with copious amounts of potassium broth taken in between produce brilliant results. Initially you may find the condition worsens as uric acid floods into the bloodstream but don't panic, keep at it. Leave at least an eight-week break between fasts, going back to a recommended vegan diet in between. I have used the seven-day deep tissue cleanse with wonderful results on arthritic and rheumatic patients. This involves seven consecutive days of fasting on organic juices, a daily colonic, vigorous skin brushing, hydrotherapy and deep body work.

HYDROTHERAPY

Repeated hot and cold showers and skin brushing to stimulate the circulation should be carried out morning and evening. If you are too poorly to do it yourself get somebody to do it for you. Take Epsom salt baths weekly (see page 47). Massaging painful joints under water using baking powder is also helpful. Movement under water in a warm swimming pool is useful too, but shower off well afterward because the chlorine in the baths is not beneficial. Paraffin wax baths are also helpful but these generally need to be administered for you and are available in naturopathic clinics.

MASSAGE OIL

A daily massage will soothe and help mobility.
Equal parts of:
St John's wort
marigold
arnica
cayenne
olive oil.
This is an excellent combination of oils.

BAREFOOT WALKING

If you are able, take a barefoot walk on grass while it is still wet with dew in the early morning. This grounds the static electricity in your body and helps to regenerate your energy. If you can't walk get someone to massage your feet daily with olive oil mixed with 10 drops of cayenne oil. After barefoot walking, dry the feet vigorously with a rough towel and get straight back into warm footwear.

EXERCISE

Do some yoga daily or, if this is currently beyond you, do some simple stretching exercises or ask a physiotherapist to work out a pattern of individual exercises for you.

RELAXATION AND VISUALIZATION

One of the common denominators I have observed among people suffering from rheumatic or arthritic disease is that they tend to be those that lavish time and attention on other people but focus very little on self-care. Rheumatism and arthritis are closely bound up with stress, the type of stress that results from the exhaustion of the adrenal glands, and conscious relaxation will help to combat this. Visualization is simply the conjuring up of graphic mental pictures which gradually works toward correcting the negative mental aspects of any disease. Read Carl Simonton's *Getting Well Again* (published by Bantam). This will help you construct a visualization programme appropriate for your own needs.

HERBS FOR ARTHRITIS SUFFERERS

Equal parts of:
white willow bark
meadow sweet flowers
wild lettuce
wild yam
black cohosh
cayenne pepper
celery seeds
wormwood.
Take 50 drops of the tincture three or four times a day as a good general remedy for arthritis.

POULTICES AND COMPRESSES

Mustard packs, castor oil compresses, clay poultices, slippery elm poultices with lobelia and cayenne added, and pulped cabbage leaf are all helpful, as long as the joint is not currently inflamed. If joints are inflamed, swelling can be reduced by eating a slice of pawpaw three times a day before each meal. Alternatively take eight tablets of digestive enzymes made from pineapple and pawpaw (available from Biocare – see Resources Directory).

PAIN RELIEF

Acupuncture can be extremely effective in relieving the pain of arthritis.

ASTHMA

The aetiology of asthma is complex. Asthma needs professional treatment and careful supervision.

In general terms, the advice outlined under hay fever is useful for asthma. Also check that there is no mould sensitivity and that all damp patches and mildew in the house are eradicated. Animal fur and feathers can sometimes makes asthma worse, so if there is a pet in the house it is important that the asthmatic avoid physical contact with it and that it should never enter the bedroom. Mattresses and carpets need to be vacuumed thoroughly once or twice a week. Many asthmatics have consistently low blood sugar and it is interesting to note that diabetics, who have high blood sugar, hardly ever have asthma. The dietary programme to follow, therefore, is one for hypoglycaemics (see page 177). Because chronic manganese deficiency may be one of the contributing causes of asthma, ensure that the diet is rich in peas, beans, blueberries, nuts and buckwheat, all of which are high in manganese.

Dry skin brushing (page 87), together with the seven hot/cold showers each morning and evening (page 50), is helpful, as are periodic juice fasts under supervision and deep breathing exercises several times a day. For acute attacks lobelia can be used under supervision and any eliminative channels which are weak or labouring need individual treatment. The following general formulation can be used in conjunction with this treatment, but is not powerful enough to help alone.

ASTHMA FORMULA

Equal parts of:
slippery elm
comfrey
marshmallow
liquorice root
elecampane.
Combine the herbs together and make a decoction; drink four breakfast-size cups a day.

RAW POTATO JUICE THERAPY

Take one medium-sized organically grown potato, wash it, cut it into thin slices with the skin on and place it in a large glass of filtered water. Let the glass stand, covered, overnight. In the morning drink the water on an empty stomach. Alternatively, freshly juice the potato and drink it diluted 50/50 with water first thing in the morning.

Many asthmatics are also hypoglycaemic or have spinal lesions as the result of injury or trauma during birth; many were weaned far too early on to excessive quantities of wheat and dairy products and received suppressive treatments for previous acute diseases, particularly eczema.

Hypoglycaemia has been linked with many allergies and asthma and can be the result of consuming an excessive amount of refined carbohydrates or stress-related adrenal malfunction. The adrenal glands are key to the glandular imbalances found with asthma. In my experience I have found spinal lesions in nearly all cases of asthma that I have treated, usually from the lower cervical to the mid-thoracic vertebrae.

Wheat and dairy products – the two most common sources of food intolerance – may upset the body's acid/alkali balance and increase the production of mucus, hence predisposing to frequent colds and other respiratory diseases. Asthmatics often have a history of chronic colds and bronchitis before the asthma itself becomes severe. I see this as the body's effort to eliminate acute diseases and if this is constantly suppressed by drug action, chronic disease much as asthma is the end result. Occasionally I have found that systemic candidiasis is a factor, and emotional insecurity plays a part too.

DIET

Again a vegan diet low in carbohydrates and with no alcohol, tea or coffee, as well as the avoidance of very hot or very cold foods and all additives in foods, helps asthma sufferers. Periods of fruit juice fasting are recommended and as many children are unable to fast, I ask children to go on a three-day all fruit diet. During acute episodes I have found a breakfast of grapefruit or grapefruit juice, fresh carrot juice at mid-morning, a lunch of plenty of steamed or baked onions and a tea of copious amounts of home-made potassium broth helpful and fast acting.

ATHEROSCLEROSIS

Hardening of the arteries, or atherosclerosis, is a common degenerative disease in which the arterial walls lose their elasticity and begin to calcify. Excessive consumption of white sugar and refined foods is one of the prime causes of hardening of the arteries, so follow the diet for heart disease (see page 173). Smoking is another contributing factor, since it affects the circulatory system (see page 222). Heavy metal toxicity may be another contributory factor and it is also vital to reduce fat in the bloodstream. Take the following steps:

- Stop smoking.
- Take moderate physical exercise. Try 40 minutes of simple walking, initially on the flat, three or four times a week building up from a few minutes to begin with and extending the time as you go along. The cumulative effect on the heart's action will soon be noticeable. A famous 19th-century Scottish doctor observed, 'I have two doctors, my left leg and my right.' Don't be frightened to use them.
- Increase foods known to help lower cholesterol and triglycerides in the blood including soya beans, tofu, legumes of all sorts, nutritional yeast, wheat, bran and oats, onions, garlic, wheatgerm, sunflower seeds, sprouted seeds of all sorts and lecithin.
- Cut out animal fats. Vitamin C deficiency may cause elevated blood cholesterol and so be one of the causes of atherosclerosis. Vitamin C helps in the conversion of cholesterol into bile acids, so make sure you have plenty of it.

- Consider coming off the contraceptive pill and hormone replacement therapy if you are on either. The Framingham study showed that HRT does not prevent heart disease or osteoporosis and actually increases the risk of breast and endometrial cancer, as well as gall bladder disease.

TONIC TO COMBAT ATHEROSCLEROSIS

One French herbalist used daily hand and foot baths of garlic and hawthorn berries equally mixed.
Alternatively, mix together the following finely powdered herbs:
Three parts of:
red clover blossom
One part of:
garlic
cayenne
ginger.
Take four capsules three times a day.

I have had patients dramatically reduce their cholesterol levels by following the advice listed and in addition taking one heaped teaspoon of cayenne in orange juice three times a day (begin with a small dose and work your way up).

CHOLESTEROL AND ITS SIGNIFICANCE

While most people are aware of the harmful effects of cholesterol in heart disease, it has now been proved that only rancid cholesterol actually causes coronary heart disease. Pure cholesterol does not. The obvious conclusion is that it is the harmful effects of rancid oil, rather than simply cholesterol, which are the primary factor. The combination of sugar or refined carbohydrates and saturated fats causes the highest increase of cholesterol and triglycerides in the blood. Our saturated fat consumption has only increased by 10% over the last 100 years whereas our consumption of refined sugar and carbohydrates has increased by 700% over the same period of time. Rancid cholesterol is likely to be present in foods which have not been stored properly, particularly pre-prepared cake, pastry and biscuit mixes.

Most people fail to understand that cholesterol is in fact made in every part of the body except the brain. While a dietary intake of cholesterol may range from 200 to 800 mg daily, the body will produce 2 g. Cholesterol is vital for the cell membrane structure, bile formation, vitamin D synthesis and steroid hormone production.

Any fats that are ingested have to be transported from the intestine to the liver where they can be metabolized. It takes several hours before they are cleared from the blood and, if the level of cholesterol remains high, any excess is deposited on the linings of the arteries, so narrowing them. Fats are transported in the bloodstream in a protein–fat compound, lipoprotein. Low-density lipoproteins are found around cholesterol-laden molecules, and when they are present in elevated levels in the bloodstream there is a higher risk of coronary heart disease. High-density lipoproteins are smaller, with more protein and less cholesterol; when high levels of these are found in the bloodstream they actually reduce the risk of coronary heart disease. The cholesterol to high-density lipoprotein ratio is vital in the battle against heart disease.

Vitamin C has a beneficial effect upon blood fats, especially cholesterol, and it reduces platelet stickiness. Anyone at risk of heart disease needs upward of 500 mg of vitamin C a day. Vitamin B complex helps keep cholesterol from collecting as plaque. Vitamin E is known to correct various platelet abnormalities and works especially well with selenium; the dosage of both needs to be individually determined. Evening primrose oil has far-reaching effects on prostaglandin metabolism. Lecithin significantly lowers blood cholesterol levels and is available in capsule form or in granules.

Oat bran fibre and oats increase high-density lipoproteins and reduce blood cholesterol, while finely powdered alfalfa works in much the same way as bran. Garlic and onions have a wonderful effect on blood fats as well as on platelet stickiness. The bromelain found in pineapple and pawpaw has beneficial effects on platelet stickiness. Ginger (preferably fresh although powdered will do) reduces platelet stickiness. Acidophili, the benign bacteria found in the digestive tract, will also lower cholesterol levels.

Sweating therapy such as Turkish baths and saunas will help exude cholesterol through the skin but the maximum amount of cholesterol is exuded with rigorous aerobic exercise. An excellent formulation for reducing cholesterol in the bloodstream is three parts red clover blossom, one part garlic, one part cayenne. All herbs should be finely powdered. Take one level teaspoon in juice morning and evening.

ATHLETE'S FOOT SEE CANDIDIASIS

BACK PAIN

This is a general term for any pain in the back, which is often symptomatic of deep organic defects. Back pain is as a direct result of kidney and bladder weakness in many instances because the toxins which are generally eliminated through the kidneys and bladder are deposited in surrounding areas of tissue, particularly the spinal joints of the lumbar region. If back pain is coupled with inflammation, nerves may become irritated resulting in sciatica, or shooting pains down the legs. Occasionally the problem can be the result of reproductive malfunction, rheumatism or back lesions.

The cause of the pain must be ascertained in order to determine whether herbs, osteopathy or acupuncture (usually the three most successful approaches) is the appropriate treatment. Often a warm and stimulating liniment will help. I have had very good results in my own clinic with my deep heat tissue massage oil but it is too complex and difficult to make at home.

COMPRESS FOR BACK PAIN

Try the following fomentation:
Two parts of:
comfrey root
marshmallow
One part of:
dandelion
ginger.
Make a decoction and soak a cloth in the strained mixture. Wrap it around the whole trunk extending from under the armpits to the pubic bone and cover it with plastic to avoid leakage. Protect the sheets with more plastic and retire to bed. Next morning unwrap yourself and sponge down with a half and half mixture of cider vinegar and warm water. Use this compress nightly until the attack of pain subsides and in the meanwhile cut out all stimulants to the kidneys including tea, coffee, cocoa, alcohol and salt and do the kidney flush on page 85.

Potters make an excellent herbal fluid extract for sciatica (see Resources Directory).

BAD BREATH SEE HALITOSIS

BALDNESS

Healthy hair is dependent on the amount and quality of the circulation in the scalp. Put simply if the blood and lymph supply to any hair follicle is cut off it will simply die. Baldness, or alopecia, therefore, may be the result of hormonal factors, as in male-pattern baldness, and in this instance the galea aponeurotica membrane in the scalp becomes thickened and inelastic. Consequently the scalp becomes thick and tight and circulation is cut off. With seborrhea and dandruff the follicles are clogged and suffocated by excessive oily secretions and accumulated dead cells but the result, baldness, is the same. Severe malnutrition, particularly the depletion of vitamin B complex in the diet, can also cause hair loss. During the last few months of pregnancy or for three or four months postpartum many women lose a large amount of hair, but this reverses itself within six months after the baby is born. Hair loss is common after severe illness or high fever but will usually regrow normally.

Once the hair follicle itself has died, no new hair growth is possible. Treatment should include a diet with the best possible nutritional value including foods rich in sulphur, silicon and iodine, which means plenty of onions, horseradish, garlic, watercress, mustard greens, radish, alfalfa, celery, lettuce, raw greens, carrots, seafood, kelp, sunflower seeds, pumpkin seeds, sprouted seeds, whole grains, wheatgerm, lecithin and nutritional yeast. Avoid absolutely salt, sugar, tobacco and alcohol. Sugar and salt, in particular, contribute toward dandruff and hair loss. Massage the scalp vigorously with the fingers or an electric vibrator every day for 20 to 30 minutes. For the first two to three weeks an excessive amount of hair will fall out but don't worry – these hairs should be replaced by strong healthier ones later on. Use a natural bristle hairbrush and brush the hair twice daily, stimulating the scalp with each stroke. Do slant-board exercises for a minimum of 20 minutes a day (see page 170). Avoid excessive shampooing and use only a mild olive oil shampoo every second day. Avoid prolonged mental work and mental stress which constrict the blood vessels in the scalp and impede the circulation. Nettles, alfalfa, parsley, kelp, birch leaves, fenugreek, onions and chili powder can all be used internally and a strong tea of nettles, horsetail, camomile, rosemary, sage, burdock or chaparral singularly or in a combination can be used as a hair rinse or conditioner. Rub a strong decoction of fresh or dry nettles into the scalp once a day after a preliminary wash with warm water without soap. Alternatively mix equal parts of castor oil and white iodine together and rub into the scalp vigorously, sitting in the sun for 15 minutes once daily. Patients have also told me that my deep heat oil used on alternative nights and left on all night acts as an excellent rubefacient but it must be kept away from the eyes at all costs.

BED WETTING SEE ENURESIS
BLADDER INFECTION SEE CYSTITIS
BREASTFEEDING

Breastfeeding babies encourages good facial and dental development, preventing poorly developed dental arches, palates and other facial collapses in adulthood. Breastfed babies are much less likely to suffer from eczema, allergies, infections, constipation and obesity. It has also been clearly demonstrated that women who breastfeed get breast cancer less than those who don't. Nursing stimulates the release of hormones from the pituitary gland, helps the uterus to return to its pre-pregnant size, burns off excess fatty tissue and, of course, the emotional bonding that develops between a mother and baby through breastfeeding creates a tremendous amount of love and trust.

As an extra bonus breast milk can convey natural medicine to a baby and I have treated very many young babies in this way with a great deal of success. However, women eating hormones hidden in meat, pesticides, additives and preservatives pass these on to the baby who in the first year is still very vulnerable. There are ways pregnant and nursing women can minimize this risk. The fewer dairy products, eggs and fish a woman consumes, the fewer toxic chemicals will be found in her breast milk. In 1976 the EPA analysed the breast milk of vegetarian women and discovered the levels of pesticide in their breast milk to be far less than average. A follow-up study in 1981 published in the *New England Journal of Medicine* confirmed that 'the highest levels of contamination in the breast milk of vegetarians was lower than the lowest level of contamination in non-vegetarian women. The mean vegetarian levels were only 1% or 2% as high as the average levels in the United States'. As yet, no studies have been done on the breast milk of vegan women but there is every likelihood that their milk is many times safer than even that of vegetarians.

Never nurse a baby lying flat on his or her back from the breast or the bottle. The nasal cavity and the mouth both connect to the back of the throat which leads in turn to openings in the middle ear. Flooding of these openings with any kind of liquid can result in recurring middle-ear infections, chronic nasal discharges and allergies. If you do decide to use a bottle, hold it in your hand and do not prop it against your baby's face. The pressure from the bottle leaning against the baby's mouth can deform the growing jaw and teeth. Ensure that the hole in the teat is large enough so that when the bottle is turned upside down milk drips easily from it: excessively hard sucking on a baby's part can lead to stomach distention.

Ideally you should aim to breastfeed for six months. Your baby will generally let you know if he or she is in need of more than breast milk by beginning to chew on your nipples. Most problems with sore nipples can be alleviated by correctly positioning the baby at the breast. Ensure that your nipple is centred in the baby's mouth with as much of the underside as the upper side taken in and get as much of the areola into the mouth as possible. Raspberry leaf tea helps to relax tense breasts and make them more flexible, as does massage with olive oil and comfrey ointment which is very comforting for cracked nipples.

If your toddler simply won't let go of the nipple because it gives him or her so much satisfaction and you are exhausted, you can discourage him or her by rubbing the nipple with a mixture of pennyroyal and myrrh tincture. The bitter taste will soon put the baby off without making him or her feel too upset.

BRONCHITIS

Stimulate the lymphatic system to assist elimination by administering hand and foot baths of equal parts of eucalyptus and thyme morning and evening. Apply hot ginger and mustard compresses to the chest but take care – if mustard is left in prolonged contact with the skin it can cause blistering in sensitive individuals.

Treat with fasting on juices. If you have the strength, take hot and cold alternate showers daily (see page 50). Learn how to breathe properly. Good breathing begins with good posture. Stand and sit tall and when you lie down make sure you are well stretched out. To check your posture and breathing follow the instructions on page 91.

Brisk sustained walking punctuated with plenty of short rests is the best type of exercise. If you want to go further, blow up several balloons daily. You can consciously work to improve your lung capacity while you walk: take four paces, hold your breath for a further four paces (if it feels uncomfortable, let it go) then breath out slowly with control for six paces. As you improve gradually increase the count. Swimming gently and consistently is also good but shower carefully afterward as chlorine is toxic.

BRUISES SEE WOUNDS, MINOR CUTS AND BRUISES

BULIMIA NERVOSA

Related to anorexia, this is where any food that is eaten publicly or privately is vomited up deliberately afterward. The acid from the vomit wears away the enamel on the teeth, so dental care is vital. The treatment is the same as for anorexia (see page 111).

BURNS

For first-degree burns (these affect the outer skin only and may cause redness, dryness, blistering and mild swelling) immerse the burn immediately in cold running water or rub it with ice cubes until all the pain has gone, even if the area goes quite numb. This stops blistering and modifies tissue damage better than anything else. If the burn is very mild cut the juicy leaf of an aloe vera open and apply the gelatinous contents directly to the burn. Aloe vera is a houseplant which can be readily at hand and is easy to grow (for suppliers see Resources Directory), or rub in St John's wort oil.

For second-degree burns, which involve the lower skin layers and may produce mottling, blistering or swelling, follow the same initial procedure and then spread the contents of a 1,000 IU capsule of vitamin E over the burn – use several capsules if the area is large. This will protect the skin while you prepare a paste of runny organic honey, powdered comfrey root and vitamin E oil. Spread this paste evenly about half an inch thick over the burn and leave it on. Do not attempt to peel it off. Simply apply more as the skin absorbs it and cover with gauze and a bandage. Continue to do this for a few days until all the pain and swelling have subsided. If for any reason you do have to remove it (and try to avoid this), soak it off with a warm decoction of echinacea and goldenseal in equal parts. Keep the burn out of the sun for at least a year and as soon as the skin is strong enough begin to skin brush daily. You may need to leave the poultice on for three weeks or longer. Don't worry. It is rebuilding and, ideally, shouldn't be disturbed. When done properly this treatment results in complete healing without any scars or damaged tissue and without the infection, pain and scraping of more orthodox medical treatment. As the scab forms over the burn simply feed it with more formulation which will rebuild the skin tissue. When the skin reveals itself it will be a nice bright fresh pink.

For acid burns, flush the area immediately with 1 pt (575 ml) of cold water into which you have stirred a teaspoon of bicarbonate of soda. Apply poultices of non-alcoholic witch hazel until the pain subsides and then cover with vitamin E oil, replenishing every hour. Seek medical advice immediately.

Third-degree burns, which involve the full thickness of the skin, need immediate medical supervision but taking powdered comfrey root internally will accelerate the healing. Take three or four heaped teaspoons a day. Continue soaking the area in ice-cold water on your way to hospital.

My American teacher, Richard Schulze, had such a severe burn on his hand that the hospital suggested a skin graft. Apart from being devoted to natural healing, he is aware of the exorbitant cost of American hospitalization and so chose to heal himself by fasting on a gallon (4.5 litres) of carrot juice daily and using the comfrey, vitamin E and honey poultice with a generous amount of lobelia added to it. (The initial extreme pain he tried to help by taking equal parts of valerian and wild lettuce, but he said it was not very effective.) He now has almost no scarring on his hand and a hand which is fully usable.

Even very severe burns can be treated extremely successfully with the above poultice, but refer yourself to a professional medical herbalist for this treatment.

A burned tongue may be cured by sprinkling a few grains of sugar on it and repeating as often as necessary.

CANDIDIASIS

The fungus *Candida albicans* is normally present in the vagina and mouth, and its growth is kept under control by bacteria in those organs. But if the body's immune system is compromised – by antibiotics or infection, for example – the fungus may multiply rapidly, resulting in thrush or moniliasis.

The symptoms that may accompany candidiasis include:

- alcohol intolerance
- anal itching
- recurrent cystitis
- constipation or diarrhoea
- craving for refined carbohydrates and/or alcohol
- depression
- fatigue
- fungal nail or skin infections, including athlete's foot
- hyperactivity
- hypoglycaemia
- inability to concentrate
- inflamed prostate gland
- iron or zinc deficiencies
- irritable bowel syndrome
- joint pains, with or without swelling
- muscle pains
- menstrual problems
- nettle rash and hives
- recurrent vaginal infections or oral thrush
- sensitivity to chemicals
- upper abdominal discomfort or burning
- bloating and flatulence.

The symptoms are worse in low or damp places, near new-mown lawns or raked-up leaves, or on days when the atmosphere is damp, all of which are symptoms of mould allergy. All symptoms are precipitated by antibiotics and there may be an onset of problems during or shortly after pregnancy.

For many years the yeast *Candida albicans* has been recognized as an important disease-producing micro-organism. It is most commonly encountered as oral and vaginal thrush and its main problem is its accurate diagnosis. Accurate diagnosis, particularly of deeply entrenched candida, can be done through Biolab (see Resources Directory, page 234). For candidiasis to be treated correctly on a permanent basis and eradicated, the efficiency of the immune system needs to be raised.

There are various normal physiological changes which, if present, predispose candida infection. These begin in infancy when the immune system is fragile and immature. It is possible for a baby to become infected with candida as it passes through the mother's vagina, if the vagina itself is infected. Pregnancy, as well as the use of oral contraceptives, predisposes to candidiasis. In old age, when the immune system functions less efficiently, it is possible to become run down, particularly as the result of insufficient nutrients in the diet or simply because the sufferers can no longer efficiently absorb the nutrients they eat. A lack of immunoglobulin A (an important antibody), a debilitated stomach wall producing too little hydrochloric acid and other conditions can predispose a person to chronic candidiasis.

In order to raise the level of the immune system and encourage it to function correctly, individual nutritional deficiencies must be corrected, but to cut out – as many practitioners treating this condition do – all forms of yeast simply because *Candida albicans* is regarded as a yeast is illogical. In my experience eating yeast in the diet does not contribute toward an overgrowth of *Candida albicans*. It is the eating of immune-suppressive refined carbohydrates and sugar that harries the immune system. I ensure that patients remain on a diet which is free of sugar in all its forms including, in the initial stages, even fresh fruit although vegetables, including juices, are strongly recommended. All tea, coffee, alcohol and salt are eliminated from the diet because to some degree they are immune suppressants. The recommended diet is wholefood and low carbohydrate, omitting anything which has been injected or fed antibiotics. Refined carbohydrates act as a food for candida in the gut so carbohydrate intake should be restricted to whole grains only and reduced to 2 oz (50 g) a day. One of the best antifungal foods available – which is also wonderful for creating benign bacteria in the gut – is garlic, so take a liver flush every morning, building up to three cloves of raw garlic, and add three more cloves to the rest of the dietary intake during the day. Initially avoid the whole fresh lemon in the liver flush and use carrot juice as your base. A diet which is initially 80% raw is particularly advised to revitalize the body.

Tea-tree oil is another excellent antifungal herb and can be applied in cream form externally to athlete's foot and used internally 1 teaspoon to 1 quart (1.1 litre) of water as a vaginal douche for thrush.

Orally, acidophilus can be taken to raise levels of benign vaginal flora but ensure that it is dairy free as you won't know whether a cow was injected with antibiotics before milking. The strength and efficacy of acidophilus supplements on the market vary greatly; the one that I recommend and have had particular success with is available from Biocare (see Resources Directory, page 240).

CATARACTS AND GLAUCOMA

Cataracts are now so common in the Western world that they are considered almost normal in the over-60s. However, experiments on lacto-sensitive babies and on rats have shown that cataracts are linked to the consumption of milk, sugar and saturated fat. Excess sugar proteinizes the effects of saturated fat in the body. Extreme nutritional deficiencies of protein or vitamin C have also been linked to some cataracts, as have improper calcium metabolism, hormone imbalance, diabetes, liver disease and many drugs. A generally toxic, devitalized body afflicted with spinal lesions in the upper cervical region, which cause alterations in blood and nervous supply affecting the health and integrity of the tissues involved, can result in cataracts.

The only herbal medication I know which has been used with some success with cataracts is *Senecio maritima*. This is administered as eye drops, one drop three times a day. Alternating hot and cold forceful head showers are helpful as are the Bates' eye exercises (detailed in his book *Better Eyesight Without Glasses*) together with neck exercises, warm castor oil eye packs, ice-cold eye baths where you will need to blink your eyes open and closed for up to five minutes in a container of ice-cold water twice per day and spinal manipulation to the cervical and upper thoracic region several times weekly for up to six weeks. Vitamin E and selenium deficiencies can also influence the rate of normal degeneration in the lens of the eye. To increase blood flow to the head take a teaspoon of cayenne pepper in juice three times a day.

Far too few people visit an optician regularly for a check-up. You should go throughout your life as naturally as you go to the dentist only not as often. Once every two or three years is fine unless you wear glasses or contact lenses in which case you should go once every 18 months. Beyond the age of 40 you should see an optician every year regardless of whether or not you wear glasses or contact lenses, because this is precisely the age at which glaucoma is most likely to develop. An experienced optician can spot not just cataracts or glaucoma but certain types of circulatory problems too. Statistically 4% of the over-40s develop glaucoma and large numbers suffer sight restriction or blindness as a result, yet glaucoma caught early can be treated very successfully by lowering the intraocular pressure and keeping it within normal range. Your optician will prescribe drops to do this locally in cases of chronic simple glaucoma.

FOR SIMPLE GLAUCOMA

The following formulation is a gentle systemic way to help to back up treatment by your optician.
Equal parts of:
angelica
dandelion root

figwort
gentian
agrimony
plantain
skullcap
Turkey rhubarb.
Take two capsules of the finely powdered herbs three times a day.

FOR DETERIORATING EYESIGHT

In my experience, the following eye formulation slows sight degeneration in many patients.
Two parts of:
eyebright
goldenseal root
fennel seed
One part of:
red raspberry leaves
mullein flowers
Half a part of:
cayenne pepper
Take 10 drops three times a day internally, and one, building up to three, drops in an eye bath full of purified water, bathing each eye and renewing the eye bath so as not to pass infection from one eye to the other, morning and evening. Also take a formulation called Vision Essentials, two capsules three times a day (see Resources Directory). Its major ingredient is bilberry extract.

CATARRH

Most of us think of catarrh as manifesting itself in the nose and sinuses but it can be present in any area of the body lined by mucous membranes. This embraces the whole of the digestive tract, fallopian tubes and vagina, as well as more obvious areas like the ears, nose and throat and upper lungs. Catarrh-forming foods include:

- dairy products
- eggs
- meat
- sugar
- tea and coffee
- chocolate
- refined foods (particularly refined carbohydrates)
- gluten (in wheat, oats, rye, and barley)
- potatoes, swedes, turnips, parsnips and any other starchy root vegetable.

If after cutting these out of your diet for two months no relief is experienced the problem may be the result of food intolerance and therefore a supervised restrictive diet needs to be followed.

I have found a superb way to remove catarrh from the system quickly is to fast for three to four days on grapefruit juice, together with supplements of hydrochloric acid. Also take a tablespoon of garlic syrup four times a day. Then follow a diet which eliminates all potentially catarrh-forming foods and include plenty of sprouted seeds as well as lots of onions, garlic, nettles and seaweed.

EXTERNAL AIDS

Fennel oil used in a vaporizing herbal bath will help to loosen mucus causing it to degenerate; the eliminative process can then remove it through the bloodstream far more easily than coughing, sneezing or blowing the nose do. This process is accelerated by the high mineral content of fennel. Simply add 10 drops of fennel oil to 1 pint (575 ml) of freshly boiled water and use this as a facial steam.

CHILBLAINS

Chilblains are the result of poor circulation, and may be the end result of an impaired blood supply because of the narrowing of the arteries. If the skin is not broken, hot mustard foot baths followed by cold dips are very helpful. Put your feet into the hot mustard bath for three minutes and then dip them quickly for 10 seconds into cold water. Repeat this routine eight times, if necessary replenishing the hot water while doing so. Use a tablespoon of mustard powder to a bucket of hot water. The soak should reach right up to the knee. Dry the feet briskly afterward with a rough towel and massage with equal parts of tincture of benzoin and camphor. Persistent and regular hot and cold foot baths will restore the circulation to normal again.

When I first arrived in the UK at the age of 14 from a tropical African climate straight into the depths of a Welsh winter, I had chilblains so badly I could barely walk. I helped myself by walking barefoot on an even stretch of snow increasing the time I could do this up to three minutes. I kept myself well covered except for my feet and then dried them once indoors by rubbing them well with my hands, then putting them straight into warm socks made of natural fibre. This radical solution worked extremely well (and was far less radical than the Romans who used to stimulate their frozen limbs while manning Hadrian's Wall by flogging themselves with nettles).

Marigold cream is excellent for soothing chilblains.

If the chilblains are broken soak them in a warm infusion of dried marigold flowers, then cover with a poultice of strained out petals: keep them in place with a bandage. This relieves the agony of broken chilblains extremely quickly and accelerates their healing. Once the skin has healed apply marigold cream or ointment.

CHILDHOOD DISEASES

CHICKENPOX

This is a viral disease which is usually mild and is characterized by crops of thin-walled vesicles which erupt and crust. Each lesion lasts two to four days, leaving a pink scar which later disappears. Pock marks may remain. Seek professional medical advice.

Give the child a warm catnip tea enema. Herbal tea such as catnip and peppermint, pleurisy root and catnip, raspberry leaf, yarrow or pennyroyal, elder-flowers and peppermint, boneset and yarrow and echinacea will all induce sweating.

Only give a child an enema under qualified supervision.

It is essential to avoid pock scarring. Try first to encourage the child not to scratch. Sponge the skin with herbal teas made as a double strength decoction of burdock root, goldenseal, or goldenseal and yellow dock root in case of severe itching. Ice-cold witch hazel is also helpful dabbed directly on to the skin with a piece of cotton cloth. Afterward dab the area dry and pat with a little arrowroot.

High doses of vitamin C have been known to help a number of viral infections including measles, mumps, shingles and chickenpox. Give a dose that takes the child just short of diarrhoea. Soluble vitamin C is usually more readily accepted.

Biochemic tissue salts are very helpful for treating children and I particularly like ferrous phosphate because it assists in the oxidation of toxins. These are available from chemists. Ask your local chemist about the appropriate dosage.

MEASLES

This begins with flu-like symptoms and also includes a cough, conjunctivitis and difficulty looking at light. It is caused by an acute viral infection and is most common in babies from six months up to five years. The temperature will fall after a day or two and then rise again suddenly by day five or six. Most noticeable with this rise is a blotchy rash which appears first on the forehead and behind the ears and rapidly spreads to the trunk; this gradually fades after three to four days. Complications may include loss of hearing, broncho-pneumonia and, very rarely, encephalomyelitis with convulsions and, extremely rarely, death. It is important to seek professional medical advice.

If you are uncertain as to the nature of the illness, take a look at the mucous membranes on the inside of the cheeks near the molars at the back. If it is a case of measles you will discover, a day or two before the blotchy rash appears on the forehead and behind the ears, that there are bright red spots with small white dots approximately ⅛ in (3 mm) in diameter. This is an unmistakable sign of measles.

Hot ginger chest poultices applied in the initial stages of the disease will bring out the rash. Then apply hot compresses of wild thyme to the skin directly to draw out internal toxins. Do not overfeed, which may lead to complications including otitis media – a middle ear infection – and broncho-pneumonia. Vitamin C needs to be taken to a point just short of diarrhoea.

To ensure oral hygiene if the child is tiny, wrap a clean cloth around your fingertip, dip it into diluted whey-concentrate and disinfect the gums and mucous membranes in the tongue which are nearly always furred. A small toothbrush dipped in the same solution can be used for bigger children.

A tea of equal parts of yarrow, pleurisy root and lady's slipper should be given to produce perspiration. It may be given freely.

Keep the room dark so that the eyes will not become irritated. If the child's eyes do become sore bathe them two or three times a day with a solution of freshly made and well-strained tea of equal parts of eyebright, raspberry leaf and goldenseal. If the child is hyperactive or irritable give camomile tea freely. If itching is a problem treat the skin as for chickenpox. If the glands become swollen give a tea of equal parts of marigold and cleavers, the dosage according to age. Also apply mullein and lobelia compresses externally as required.

The biotissue salt Kali-phosphate will help if there is any suggestion of lung or bronchial complications (ask your chemist about the dose). A tincture of sundew is useful if a cough develops (again dosage according to age).

MUMPS

This is an acute viral infection characterized by a low fever, lassitude and a sore throat with swollen parotid glands. You should seek professional medical advice. Swelling may occur unilaterally or bilaterally. Although the fever usually only lasts for a few days, the swelling can go on for weeks. Complications are extremely rare before puberty, but involve swelling of the ovaries or testicles which may affect later reproductive ability.

Treat as for chickenpox in terms of diet and bed rest. Treat swollen glands internally and externally with mullein and lobelia formulation. Replace the external compress every half hour during the day and leave on all night.

Administer warm sitz-baths, adding equal parts of an infusion of arnica and marigold to the water.

Particularly painful testicles will benefit from a warm poultice of St John's wort oil or whey concentrate. Ensure the feet are kept warm while the poultices are applied. If a girl is complaining of stomachache, administer an appropriate dose of pulsatilla every second hour while awake. The adult dose is one size 0 capsule: adjust according to age.

Gargling with whey concentrate or a tincture of thyme will soothe sore throats. In all cases give the following formulation in addition to other suggested remedies: two parts echinacea, one part ginseng (Siberian), one part goldenseal, one part yellow dock and half a part ginger root. For children under 10, substitute angelica root for the ginseng.

Of the finely powdered herbs, in the case of teenagers and adults take four size 0 capsules twice daily until completely recovered, including the period of convalescence but for not longer than three weeks in all. Alter the dose accordingly for children. Take no coffee while on this remedy.

WHOOPING COUGH

This is one of the most serious childhood diseases and treatment should be particularly vigorous and consistent to get the best results. It is important to consult a qualified medical herbalist. Whooping cough is an acute bacterial infection characterized by severe paroxysmal coughing. The bacteria grows on the trachea and bronchi producing an endotoxin which sensitizes nerve endings in the respiratory tract, and may have a toxic effect on the central nervous system. Symptoms include a mild fever, flu-like symptoms and a cough followed by a sudden whooping sound as breath is taken in. This may also cause vomiting. Paroxysms are usually worse at night and the disease can go on for two to four weeks, or more. Complications include convulsions, bleeding from the nose or broken blood vessels in the sclera or – more seriously – into the brain, and broncho-pneumonia.

Keep the child warm and in bed. Fast on fruit juice, especially pineapple and citrus, for a few days then introduce potassium broth, vegetable juices and fresh fruit. Overfeeding makes the condition worse.

Apply a garlic foot compress and chest poultices of onion, horseradish or mustard. Take care that they do not blister the skin by overlong contact. Maximum reddening of the skin shows the poultice should be removed. Steam inhalation of Olbas oil (available at all pharmacies) will also help.

TO SOOTHE WHOOPING COUGH

Equal parts of:
bayberry
hyssop
raspberry leaves
Turkey rhubarb
thyme.
Decoct the first four herbs then put this over the thyme and infuse for half an hour,
covered. Strain. Take one teaspoon or more as needed, depending on age.

GENERAL

Regard children's diseases as beneficial in so far as fevers involve disposal of pathological material within the system that would otherwise cause more serious conditions later on. Provided the child is healthy, the disease will easily be overcome and the body strengthened as a result of doing so. It is essential to ensure that all childhood diseases are treated properly and not suppressed. Fevers destroy not only the poisons accumulated during the lifetime of the child, they also eliminate many of those toxins which have been brought over from the embryonic stage of development. In my experience people who have never had any childhood ailments are apt to succumb to all sorts of diseases later in life. Properly handled fevers are curative in as much as they protect us from, rather than expose us to, diseases. Also having properly endured a childhood disease we tend not to get it twice because we build up antibodies to it.

Childhood fevers escalate quickly and, if left untreated, can cause convulsions. Get help if you are in any doubts as to the severity of your child's illness.

Diet is the single most important factor that protects us from or disposes us to childhood diseases. Give a germ lots of soil to flourish on and it will wreak all kinds of havoc; in this case, soil means sugar and other refined carbohydrates. I have no patience with parents who complain that a sick child will not eat green vegetables. Wean a baby on to green vegetables and fresh fruits, leaving the unprocessed cereals, especially wheat, till last and you should have no problems. A well-fed child will develop a strong, healthy reaction to any childhood disease and get over it quickly. It is far better to develop a short-term high fever with a good rapid rash development and heavy sweating than a mild fever, light perspiration, and a nearly invisible rash.

TREATMENT

Basic treatment for most childhood infections is simple. Nearly all children who are left to their own instincts will ask for only liquids, so offer only fruit and vegetable juices, home-made lemonade (with no added sugar), plenty of mineral water and herbal tea.

Work with the fever by applying warm packs to the body using either compresses or poultices over the infected areas. Warm baths are also helpful. In both instances such gentle hydrotherapy encourages perspiration which is essential. The bowels must be kept open and working freely, so herbal laxatives or small rectal injections of lukewarm herbal teas may be needed. The best ones to administer are catnip, camomile or horsetail. Rectal injections consist of only 5 fl oz (150 ml) of liquid.

Do not attempt to administer an enema to a child without supervision from a qualified medical herbalist.

CIRRHOSIS OF THE LIVER

The functions of the liver are enormously diverse. Not only is it one of the largest organs in the body but it acts as the body's laboratory. It stores energy in the form of glycogen. It generates energy as glucose from the amino acids and fatty constituents that we absorb via our food, and processes protein, not merely by taking proteins apart but by also synthesizing new ones. The liver is the connecting link between the proteins of the animal and plant kingdoms and human protein. It also acts as a central station for detoxification, both of foreign poisons and those produced by the body itself. Additionally bilirubin (a by-product of the decomposition of the red pigment of blood, haemoglobin) has to be changed in the liver into a form that can be excreted. If this process is interrupted it leads to jaundice. Finally, the liver synthesizes urea which is excreted by the kidneys. So vital is the health of the liver that many natural therapists feel that the recovery from cancer depends directly on the degree of damage to liver function. While every other part of the body can and does regenerate itself in less than a year, the liver has an extraordinary capacity to do so very quickly, so partial destruction may be restored fairly rapidly providing the deterioration is not extensive and rapid. Conversely the liver can remain damaged for a long time before the deterioration is detected, so that its great functional reserves are exhausted. It is here that iridology comes into its own as a diagnostic tool because it is so useful in evaluating the exact degree of degeneration.

Liver cirrhosis is generally, but by no means always, the result of excessive consumption of alcohol. Low levels of nickel occur in people with cirrhosis. The herbal approach to cirrhosis is a long-term one using herbs which act directly on the liver, increasing the flow of bile, as well as bitter herbs which promote digestion. These need to be chosen selectively according to individual need by a fully qualified medical herbalist.

COELIAC DISEASE

This is an inability to digest the gluten in wheat, oats, rye and barley. It can begin at any age and manifests itself as diarrhoea, colic, bloating, what is loosely but incorrectly called irritable bowel syndrome, depression, infertility, or a variety of gut upsets. It is essential to have a correct diagnosis by a specialist as gluten intolerance is also possible even if the small intestinal lining is shown to be healthy. It is also possible to be allergic to wheat without being intolerant of gluten.

Should a diagnosis be confirmed there are some excellent books on gluten-free cookery on the market.

The first step is to avoid all gluten products. Ground brown rice and carrot juice mixed together as a gruel will help children with coeliac disease.

Apply abdominal compresses of camomile and take warm sitz-baths of camomile daily. Use herbs which are high in mucilage to soothe the lining of the intestine. Slippery elm, comfrey root or marshmallow are helpful. These can be mixed to a thick paste and eaten off the spoon directly or thinned with more liquid to a gruel and drunk a cup at a time.

....

The ingestion of large amounts of comfrey root needs to be done under the supervision of a qualified medical herbalist.

....

However marshmallow and slippery elm may be taken freely.

COLD SORES

A cold sore is a small blister that, when ruptured, leaves a thin yellowish crust often exacerbated by broken skin which bleeds or weeps. It is the result of a viral infection which can be sparked off by rubbing or chafing the skin, injury, physical or mental strain, sunburn, fever, poor diet, excessive anger, anxiety, depression and menstruation. Certain people have regular outbreaks of cold sores while others seem relatively immune even when exposed. Overall, the common denominator seems to be a condition of immune deficiency attached to stress or dietary indiscretions, with local irritation as an instigating factor. Hence raising the level of the immune system is an essential prerequisite as is a dietary strategy which involves the reduction of the amino acid arginine and the simultaneous boosting of lysine which helps to control duplication of the viral particles. Foods rich in lysine include beans, nutritional yeast and bean sprouts, as well as fruits and most vegetables except peas. Foods high in arginine are gelatin, chocolate, coconut, oats, whole wheat or white flour, wheatgerm, peanuts and soya beans.

To raise the level of the immune system, dry skin brush daily and take the kind of aerobic exercise which acts as a powerful pump for the lymph glands (you have your choice between swimming, trampolining, brisk walking, running and skipping). Echinacea is a particularly useful herb for the lymph system as it assists the production of white blood cells and is a supreme lymph cleanser, so keep yourself, if your immunity is low, on a regular dose of 15 drops of the tincture three times a day. Foods which clog up the lymph system include meat, dairy products, sugar, anything artificial, alcohol and fried foods.

At the first signs of tingling apply ice for up to 20 minutes, then dab on a lotion of equal parts of garlic, goldenseal and skullcap. Repeat this routine frequently throughout the day. If the skin becomes scabby alternate with aloe vera cream or vitamin E oil.

There is now an excellent lip salve called Vy-Brite available in many chemists and health-food shops which is based on oil of melissa and which, if used regularly morning and evening, acts as an excellent preventative against cold sores. It is therefore particularly useful for people who are especially predisposed to them.

COLDS

A cold that is properly managed should last for only two or three days and flow purposely and freely. If you are in good health, colds are rare. Any cold that is discouraged and suppressed may drag itself on one way or another for several months.

Zinc lozenges (which are suckable) have been shown to shorten the duration of symptoms of the common cold.

A well-known herbal remedy for colds is equal parts of an infusion of elderflowers, peppermint and yarrow. Have a hot bath while drinking 1 pint (575 ml) of this (sweeten if necessary with honey and lemon), then dry yourself vigorously, get into cotton nightwear, go to bed, cover yourself with plenty of warm bedclothes and settle down to have a good sweat. While awake in bed, assist the eliminative function of a cold with plenty of ginger tea with honey, lemon, a pinch of cayenne pepper and a crushed clove of garlic in each mug. Hot mustard foot baths will decongest the head and salt water douches into the nose using a nasal spray will decongest the sinuses. Facial steam inhalation using essential oils of eucalyptus, thyme, cloves or the combination of oils in Olbas oil are helpful too. If a sore throat is the problem, spray echinacea tincture liberally directly down the throat. Not only is this antiviral and antibacterial, but in this form it also has the ability to stop soreness by numbing it.

Fasting on fruit juice for two to three days also helps. The old adage correctly worded is if you feed a cold you will then have to starve a fever so eating during a cold is not a good idea. Take juice and plenty of mugs of ginger tea. Don't fast for longer than three days, which may prolong the cold. Instead go on a diet which includes plenty of onions, garlic and citrus fruit.

COLIC

Colic is believed to be related to the amount of air ingested by a baby during feeding, and is less common among babies who are breastfed than bottle-fed unless they are being upset by something the mother is eating. Onions, garlic, wheat, yeast and green leafy vegetables are the most usual culprits. Colic is also found in babies who pick up on the high stress levels of the mother. Bottle-fed babies who show signs of colic may be intolerant of milk, soya milk or sugar in formula feeds. The alternative is diluted goat's milk or better still rice, oat or nut milk.

....

Discuss any change in feeding an infant under three months with a qualified health professional.

....

True colic is very rare after a baby is three months old. Look to wheat intolerance as the culprit: children can only digest wheat really well after the first year.

INFANTILE COLIC FORMULA

An excellent formula for infantile colic is an infusion of equal parts of catnip and fennel. Give two teaspoons every 10 minutes, or as often as needed. Apply a warm compress of peppermint to the stomach. Alternatively, the mother who is breastfeeding a baby can take one teaspoon of wild yam tincture every three hours.

CONJUNCTIVITIS

This occurs when the eye becomes red, gritty, watery and painful. Its vernal form, this is the type that frequently occurs in the spring, is more often than not due to calcium deficiency.

It is widely believed that dairy products are the best and most effective source of calcium but in fact plants are by far the best assimilated form of calcium. Pint for pint carrot juice contains more calcium than milk. Fast for three days using carrot juice and Superfoods and assist the kidneys during the fast with dandelion tea. Decoct cornflower, mullein, plantain, marigold, eyebright, fennel, liquorice, camomile or raspberry leaves (infusions may not sterilize the herbs adequately in this instance). Bathe the eyes often with one of these decoctions ensuring that it is well strained and reheat it so that it is lukewarm before use. Take 10 drops of goldenseal tincture before each meal as long as the condition lasts and then discontinue.

Vitamin B_2 deficiency manifests as a red ring around the front of the eye so do not get the two muddled. Food allergies can sometimes cause repeated conjunctivitis so if this is a problem it may be worth having it investigated.

CONSTIPATION

Chronic constipation is the result of a variety of physiological and psychological factors including:

- liver malfunction (especially gall bladder disease)
- underactive thyroid function
- appendectomy
- anaemia
- addiction to laxatives
- specific food intolerance
- constant worry/depression
- refusing to go to the toilet to defecate when you have a natural urge to do so
- a low-fibre diet with too much animal protein, resulting in putrefaction in the colon
- vitamin and mineral deficiencies, particularly vitamin C and magnesium
- diverticular disease
- not drinking enough liquids regularly; ideally an adult should drink a minimum of 7 pints (4 litres) daily
- irritable bowel syndrome
- drugs and substances that affect bowel mobility (opiates, iron tablets, certain anti-depressants, antacids)
- long periods of immobility; this particularly applies to the elderly
- painful anal conditions that inhibit the opening of the bowels
- spinal lesions

- prolapsed colon
- partial intestinal obstructions, such as adhesions and cancer
- absence of normal nerve plexus and ganglia on the wall of the colon – a condition which is extremely rare.

Overall, poor diet plays the largest part in constipation. The bowel should dump literally pounds of waste every day. Most people get rid of 8–10 oz (225–285 g) and think they are doing well, even if they have up to three bowel movements daily, but in truth everyone should eliminate four-fifths of the food they ingest over a 10–18 hour period. It is possible to conduct a rather novel experiment to find out if this is so by liquidizing the entire intake of food for a day, taking a long hard look at it and seeing if most of this emerges at the other end.

Check to see how long food takes to pass through the body. It is not uncommon for people to retain faeces for days. Do this with the sunflower seed test. Eat a heaped handful of sunflower seeds, chewing as little as possible, and time their passage through the colon. They will show up very clearly, white and grey, in the faeces. (Sunflower seeds are high in vitamin F which helps to rebuild the mucous lining of the colon, so eating them plentifully and chewing them well under normal circumstances helps.) A sluggish colon is just as dangerous as an impacted one. The prolonged retention of faeces can be one of the sources of heart disease because a poisonous bloodstream raises cholesterol in the blood serum alarmingly, predisposing the body to coronary disease. The chemical changes to the bile produced by retention may also be responsible for tumours and cancer.

A prolapsed colon and rectal problems can be dealt with by learning to defecate properly and by slant-board exercises (see page 170). Squatting is the best position to adopt when defecating. In so-called less civilized countries this position with thighs flexed against the abdomen ensures the stomach muscles are provided with the support they need. Western WCs do not suit the physiology of the body. They are too high to allow for a squatting position and the sitting-on-a-chair posture they encourage is essentially passive and unable to assist the body's mechanism. In addition, Western clothing actively impedes a squatting position.

Sit on the toilet with your arms crossed at the chest and draw your feet back. Or put a small stool, a box or a pile of magazines about 12 in (30 cm) high in front of the toilet to raise your feet and, if you are suffering from any internal prolapses, defecate while placing your hands on your head. This will relieve the bearing down on rectal muscles, prevent haemorrhoids and relieve the strain on upper abdominal muscles.

There are WCs designed to encourage a more healthy and comfortable position even when used on a unit of conventional height. The shape is elongated to provide comfort and room for men and curved to give thighs the support that the conventional WC lacks, but as far as I can ascertain such seats are only available in Italy.

There is a device on the market called the stool stool which acts in a similar way and can be transported (although it is about the size of a medium handbag).

THE MICROLIFE OF THE INTESTINES

A healthy colon holds 3–4 lb (1.3–1.8 kg) of resident bacteria as indigenous flora. Such flora is composed of 300–400 different species of bacteria whose activities affect our metabolism, physiology and biochemistry in ways both beneficial and harmful. So vital is this intestinal metabolic activity that it even exceeds the liver in the wide range of its metabolic processes. A constipated colon has a much higher proportion of abnormal bacteria in it with a consequently greater potential for cancer.

The bacterioids, together with coliform bacilli and *E. coli*, are the putrefactive bacteria responsible for the decaying matter in the colon. They prefer a diet full of protein and fat which accelerates the output of undesirable metabolites like bile salts, urea, phenols, ammonia and other dietary degradation products which are all potentially harmful substances, doubly so if there is constipation or impaired detoxification by the liver. A high population of poor bacteria is one of the main contributory factors in the development of all sorts of degenerative diseases like ulcerative colitis, diverticulitis, haemorrhoids and colonic cancer and most people have a ratio of 85% of these potentially harmful bacteria to only 15% beneficial bacteria.

The 15% beneficial bacteria produce acetic, lactic and formic acid which lower the pH of the intestine and so prevent the colonization of fungi like *Candida albicans* (which causes thrush). When the percentage is better balanced, with 75% of these beneficial bacteria, peristalsis is stimulated, flushing out toxic bacterial metabolites and waste products in the faeces, so checking putrefactive bacteria. It is possible to alter this balance with a thorough bowel cleanse coupled with supplementations of acidophilus (for suppliers see Resources Directory) and a healthy lacto-vegetarian diet.

It is quite common for the elderly, who generally have a tired, worn-out stomach lining resulting in achlorhydria (under-secretion of hydrochloric acid), to have too many of the bacterioids. Achlorhydria is also the result of consuming too much tannic acid in tea and coffee (yet another good reason to give them up) or of taking very hot or cold drinks or foods as well as indulging in high-fat, high-protein diets which favour meat. Benign bacteria flourish in lacto-vegetarian diets high in fibre and whole grains.

Breastfeeding leads to a flora with a predominance of benign bacteria. During the process of birth the baby is exposed to micro-organisms from the mother's vagina and intestinal tract and afterward obtains these from the environment from being handled. The bacteria which colonized the skin and the mucosal surfaces of the upper respiratory and gastro-intestinal tracts mark the beginning of a lifelong symbiosis between the human organism and the indigenous flora.

Bottle-fed babies have a much high density of bacterioids, clostridia and *Lactobacillus acidophilus* with few benign bacteria. Breastfed babies have acidic stools with a pH ranging from 5–5.5 which increases their capacity to resist infection by pathogenic bacteria. Bottle-fed babies have a faecal flora closer to those of adults in its consistency and odour with a pH of 6–7. So breast milk clearly comes out tops as far as healthy bacteria are concerned, as well as having other immunological properties. Breastfed babies maintain a stronger component of benign bacteria as they grow up than their bottle-fed cousins. It seems that breastfeeding is the first and most vital factor in the balance of desirable bacteria in the colon.

ENCOURAGING BENEFICIAL BACTERIA

It is possible to balance your intestinal bacteria by eating lots – 12 fl oz (350 ml) – of live yogurt daily. Anything added to the yogurt except a well-ripened banana will destroy much of the benign bacteria in it, so it must be eaten plain. Bananas, provided they are well ripened (the way to tell is to choose those with brown freckles all over their skins), are the only fruit known actively to encourage the growth of beneficial flora in the colon.

The problem with both bananas and yogurt for some people is that they create a lot of mucus and 12 oz (350 ml) of yogurt is a lot to get through in one sitting. The alternative is to take acidophilus, a freeze-dried form of benign lactobacilli. There are many other forms of acidophilus on the market but I have found bioacidophilus to be infinitely superior (see Resources Directory).

If overgrowth of the yeasts and fungal colonies in the intestines is the problem, an Argentinean tree bark called pau d'arco has long been used by the Inca Indians in Southern Peru to introduce a whole spectrum of complex biochemical properties based on its active ingredient lapachol into the intestine. Drink two cups of pau d'arco tea daily for its fungicidal properties (there is much ersatz pau d'arco tea on the market so do check that you are buying the real thing).

The regulatory activity of faecal microflora has been shown to have a greater effect on bowel function than the addition of dietary fibre. It is not uncommon for me to encounter patients who have been eating vast amounts of bran, to achieve nothing other than an irritable bowel and lots of flatulence. Acidophilus improves transit time through the gastro-intestinal tract, which prevents auto-intoxication ('self-poisoning'). Eli Metchnikoff, the first person to appreciate the medical benefits of fermented milk, observed, 'Not only is the auto-intoxication from the microbial poisons absorbed in cases of constipation, but microbes themselves pass through the walls of the intestine and enter the blood.'

Constipation is the hub of the mechanism in many disease processes. Toxins and micro-organisms pass through the intestinal wall into the body, causing an endless array of disturbances. The body then absorbs poisons from the waste decaying in the colon and the end result is self-poisoning. Meat, fish and eggs provide the most harmful metabolites, which on entering the bloodstream create a toxic load for the cells throughout the body and in particular the liver. This self-poisoning causes fatigue, poor concentration, irritability, insomnia, headaches and muscular aches, and leads to degenerative diseases.

BRAN

One of the things recommended by doctors for constipation is to increase fibre in the diet and stop refined carbohydrate foods. One of their favourite prescriptions is wheat bran, which is not necessarily the best solution. Not only are many people wheat intolerant, but if you look at wheat bran under a microscope it has claws on it almost like thorns and these can dig into an already irritable mucous membrane, exacerbating the problem. Recently it was discovered that four out of every 100 blood donors had laboratory evidence of an allergy to gluten in wheat. Gluten is also present in rye, oats and barley. I prefer to prescribe rice bran or, better still, flax seed or psyllium husks, the outer seed coats of plantain. Alternatively try the laxative gruel.

LAXATIVE GRUEL

Three parts of:
comfrey root
psyllium husks or Linusit Gold (organically-grown flax seed, available in health food shops)
liquorice root
marshmallow root
Mix with fruit juice and sweeten with honey if desired. Take one tablespoon at a time or more as needed. The flax seed or psyllium husks act as bulk, the liquorice root is a mild laxative, the marshmallow root is to assist clearance where hard stools are prevalent, while the comfrey root heals and rebuilds weaker areas in the colon and gives lubrication.

If constipation is a long-standing problem, a thorough bowel cleanse is advisable. Alternatively see the formulation Intestinal Corrective No. 3 on page 152.

HERBAL COMBINATION TO AID IMPROPER BOWEL FUNCTION
INTESTINAL CORRECTIVE NO. 1

This is a unique and unbeatable formula for treating all bowel problems and is also helpful as part of the treatment for haemorrhoids. It is the aim of this formulation to restore normal bowel function, not to create a dependence as most laxatives do. A combination of herbs cleanses the liver and gall bladder, starts the bile flowing, and stimulates peristalsis so that layers of encrusted ancient mucus can gradually slough off as the bowel is rebuilt, resulting in a perfect assimilation of food. It clears out the bowel pockets and diverticula, healing any inflamed areas and relaxing any areas of tension.

Two parts of:
cascara sagrada
One part of:
bayberry bark
cayenne
fennel
goldenseal
lobelia (available only from qualified medical herbalists)
red raspberry leaves
Turkey rhubarb root.

Combine all the herbs, which should be finely powdered, and fill size 0 gelatine capsules with them. If lobelia is unavailable, substitute ginger.

DR CHRISTOPHER'S FORMULATIONS

Dr Christopher's formula produces a very individual result and therefore the dosage must be monitored and adjusted according to individual response. As there are no two people alike in age, size or physical constitution (and certainly people's bowels are as different as their fingerprints), you will have to regulate the dose according to your own needs. I would suggest that you begin by taking two capsules three times a day, with meals, or if you don't eat three times a day take two capsules with every meal that you do eat in order to achieve a bowel movement for every meal ingested. If you get diarrhoea cut down; if you can't get a bowel movement raise the dosage until you can. Some of my patients have had to take as many as 15 capsules with each meal for the first few months of this formula. This simply means the person concerned is chronically constipated and it is taking some time before the body releases its accumulated faecal matter.

The bits of encrusted mucus that emerge may look odd. You may see nuts and seeds, which have been lodged in the colon for months or even years; traces of barium meal (if you have ever had one); bits of what looks like rubber tyre, tree bark or coloured Vaseline jelly. Alternatively bowel movements may emerge smelling particularly foul or may emerge accompanied by a great deal of rumbling or flatulence. Don't be alarmed by any of this. Do not taper off the formulation so much you lose the momentum and so the continuity of this elimination. A thorough bowel cleanse for a constipated person takes from nine months to a year or longer.

It is essential to combine this gastro-intestinal cleansing with a diet which is totally free of dairy products, eggs, meat and all refined foods for at least the first six months of a bowel cleanse. It is simply a waste of effort to put items which cause constipation in one end while you continue to try and pull impacted faeces from the other.

To determine whether the process is at an end and your colon is perfectly clean, go on a carrot juice and purified water fast for a day. Try to drink at least eight large glasses of carrot juice and plenty of water. The resultant faeces should emerge looking bright orange-brown. If they are a mixture of brown and orange-brown this means there is still some old encrusted matter emerging and the process needs to be continued. If they are completely brown it means you have got a very long way to go.

Fasting for one regular day a week, together with enemas morning and evening, greatly helps this bowel-cleansing process.

....

Note: Omit the goldenseal from the bowel-cleansing formula after two months and replace it with equal parts of wild thyme and garlic. Goldenseal destroys the B vitamins if taken long term. Also, omit if you are pregnant or diabetic. This formulation should not in any case be taken for longer than one year.

....

HERBAL FORMULA FOR CHRONIC CONSTIPATION
INTESTINAL CORRECTIVE NO. 2

I occasionally label this affectionately the TNT formula and use it only when patients are chronically constipated.

Equal parts of:
agrimony
alfalfa
Cape aloe
cascara sagrada
cayenne
garlic
ginger
senna pods
wild yam root

*Combine all the herbs, which should be finely powdered, and fill size 0 gelatine capsules with them. Take one before each meal (one of these is the equivalent of four of the Intestinal Corrective No. 1s). Increase the dose by one capsule a day (**not one capsule a meal**). Continue to adjust the dose until you are having a bowel movement for every meal you eat.*

OTHER AIDS

- Take alternate hot and cold sitz-baths daily. For a spastic colon apply a hot castor oil poultice to the abdomen nightly, all night, for six consecutive nights weekly. Keep it as hot as possible with a hot water bottle at least for the first few hours.
- Fast on freshly pressed apple juice for one day regularly every week, choosing the same day each week. Take nothing else, including herbs, except mineral water, and take a warm catnip enema morning and evening on this fasting day.
- Increase abdominal strength with yoga exercises and get plenty of daily vigorous exercise every day, walking, swimming, horseriding or hill climbing.

- Visit the toilet after every meal to ingrain the reflex of opening the bowels.
- Don't drink with meals. Aim to drink seven pints of liquid daily.

CORNS

My mother used to make me wear good, sturdy, well-fitted shoes, when all I longed for, as a little girl, was those patent leather black party shoes which were flimsy and thin heeled. As an adult with excellent feet I am eternally grateful to her. Corns are often the result of incorrect footwear. Macerate 1 oz (30 g) of ivy leaves and the same quantity of celandine leaves in enough cider vinegar to barely cover, leaving it standing for a fortnight in an airing cupboard. Shake several times daily and top up with vinegar from time to time if need be. Fork out some of the leaves and bind them into the corner of a piece of liniment and bandage. Apply this to the corn and change the dressing twice daily. If you persist you will find the corn will gradually get soft enough to lift out.

Alternatively, apply a crushed clove of garlic to the corn protecting the surrounding area with olive oil or Elastoplast. Secure it with a bandage or plaster and renew this poultice once daily.

COUGHS

Take a teaspoon of syrup of garlic or 10 drops of plantain tincture in water as often as needed. The diet should be one of warm vegetable broths and soupy grains as long as the cough lasts.

COUGH MIXTURE

> If the cough is very pronounced and racks the body take this remedy.
> Equal parts of:
> comfrey root
> Icelandic moss
> mullein
> slippery elm
> wild cherry bark
> wild lettuce.
> Take a teaspoon of this tincture every second hour alternating with a teaspoon of garlic oil.

To kill the infection take 360 drops of echinacea tincture a day for 10 consecutive days. Use a ginger root compress on the chest or rub in deep heat oil.

CRABS

Most people who have crabs know from the incessant itching of pubic hair that something is awry. The eggs take from seven to nine days to hatch and each crab is capable of laying three eggs a day. Crabs are easily transmitted not only by sexual contact but by sitting on the same couch, using the same toilet, or sharing a bed with someone who has them.

To 3 fl oz (75 ml) olive oil add 10 drops each of rosemary oil and lavender oil, 12 drops of eucalyptus oil and 13 drops of geranium oil. Saturate the area infested (usually the pubic area although they can survive in any hairy part of the body) with the oil and cover with close-fitting plastic pants or wrap the area in cling-film. Leave on for two hours. Remove over the toilet and shampoo. Comb through the hair with a fine-toothed comb to remove any eggs. Repeat the treatment after three days and again after a further three days.

CRADLECAP

The flaky scalp of a newborn usually clears naturally; it may, however, be exacerbated by dairy products. If the baby is being breastfed, ensure that the mother drinks a pint of nut milk a day, eating the remaining almond sludge sieved out of the milk by adding it to soups and cereals. Ensure her intake of magnesium and B_6 is adequate. If the baby is bottle-fed, get advice on switching from a formula based on cow's milk.

Massage the baby's scalp with St John's wort oil for five minutes and then leave it on for a further half hour. Brush the scalp well, taking care not to cause bleeding or create inflammation, and then rinse out the oil with a heavily diluted natural shampoo ensuring it does not run into the eyes. Finish with a tepid rinse making sure there is no trace of shampoo left and repeat twice weekly until the condition has cleared.

CRAMPS

Nutritionally, leg cramps respond to moderately high doses of vitamin E and nutritional yeast as well as foods rich in calcium and magnesium. Occasionally food intolerance may be causing the cramps so this should be investigated.

Cramp bark tincture, one teaspoon three times a day, is very helpful for menstrual cramps. To speed its effect put it in a small amount of hot water. If the cramps are long established investigate the possibility of chronic candidiasis. Sometimes a potassium deficiency can be a major contributory factor. Restless twitching legs at night can be due to iron deficiency which may be the result of excessive menstrual bleeding or excessive tea consumption. Iron is richly present in Superfoods (see page 18).

CYSTITIS

Cystitis is a bacterial infection which inflames the bladder. It is 30 times more common in females than in males. The short female urethra and close proximity of this to the anus are predisposing factors.

AVOIDING CYSTITIS

- Drink plenty of fluid, at least 7 pints a day if possible.
- Eat food which will encourage the health of the immune system, that is, food that is 80% raw, natural and unprocessed, low in sugar, alcohol and animal fat.
- Pay special attention to personal hygiene. After a bowel movement the anus should be cleaned from front to back so that no germs are carried toward the external opening of the bladder; this also applies after urination.
- Don't use soaps, detergents and perfumed toiletries when washing the vaginal and anal areas. Plain water is good enough and running water is even better.
- Don't wear nylon underwear, tights or trousers.
- Wash the genitals before and after sex.

If none of these measures helps, ask your practitioner to check for the possibility of chronic candidiasis, and the possibility that you may be allergic to a specific food.

TREATMENT

Follow a liquid fast for five days drinking apple juice, mineral water, and three cups of cider vinegar and honey mixed with hot water during the course of the day. Potassium broth and barley water are also helpful, as is cranberry juice, because it reduces the adhesion of bacteria to the membrane walls. Include four glasses of this a day during the course of your fasting.

After the fast go on to a vegan diet ensuring that your fluid intake is still high. The bowels must be opened at least once daily to ensure that there is no possibility of retaining toxins which can be recirculated into the blood and eventually have to be handled by the kidneys.

Crouching over a wide deep bowl of steaming hot camomile and thyme infusion also helps. If this is uncomfortable place the basin underneath a chair from which you have removed the base. Surround yourself and the chair in a heavy blanket and keep as warm as possible. As the steam subsides keep topping it up with hot water. I have found this even more effective than the usual recommended hot sitz-bath for pain relief. Hot compresses of parsley root and glycerine applied to the bladder and kidneys are also helpful.

CYSTITIS TEA

Take as much as you can manage of the following tea, and not less than four cups daily:
One part of:
dandelion root
horsetail
uva ursi leaves
camomile flowers
nettles
meadowsweet flowers
Two parts of:
buchu leaves

If there is blood in the urine apply a poultice of cornsilk tassels to the kidneys and abdomen and add four parts of cornsilk to the formulation above.

DANDRUFF

Dandruff is usually the result of an incorrect diet coupled with excessive sebaceous gland activity. Some naturopaths believe there is a connection to fungal infection so it is worth checking to see if you have candidiasis.

Use an olive oil shampoo to wash the hair and massage the scalp thoroughly nightly with your fingertips using liberal applications of tincture of rosemary. Follow this with a poultice of flax seed oil, protecting the pillow case with thick towels. Wash this out well in the morning with the olive oil shampoo. Rinse the hair with a cup of cider vinegar in a basin full of water. Repeat this treatment on a nightly basis until the dandruff has completely disappeared.

DEAFNESS SEE MÉNIÈRE'S DISEASE AND TINNITUS

DEPRESSION

The mentally ill occupy as many as one-third of hospital beds. Physical causes of depression include:

- an underactive thyroid
- nutritional deficiencies
- heavy metal toxicity
- food intolerance
- hypoglycaemia
- chronic candidiasis
- endocrine imbalance.

Emotional causes of depression can include:

- isolation
- no close friends to confide in
- having no work outside the home
- poor housing
- financial problems
- looking after toddlers at home full time
- losing your mother at an early age.

The roots of depression spring from not being in control of your life. A feminist sociologist, Pauline Bart, explains depression as a response to powerlessness. She believes that women are set up for depression in society by encouraging or forcing them to 'put their eggs in one or at most two baskets – the mother role and the wife role'. When they lose one or both of these roles many women respond with a loss of identity and a sense of powerlessness and uselessness. Depression can apply equally to career women crippling themselves in the attempt to be superwomen. People who retire unwillingly are notoriously prone to depression.

- St John's wort in tincture form is excellent for treating depression. The normal adult dose is 20 drops three times a day.
- Physical exercise certainly helps, by stimulating the brain to release endorphins, the so-called happy hormones. One of the most common signs of depression is fatigue. Make your exercise regular, vigorous and enjoyable and, given time, it will revolutionize your physical and mental well-being.
- Fighting back helps. If your rights or dignity are being trampled on, summon the energy to stand up for yourself. Say what you mean. Show your feelings. Purposeful activities helps: make sure it is something you really enjoy that will give you a sense of accomplishment.
- Put in a positive context, depression can be seen not just as struggle and pain, but as an opportunity for enlightenment and growth, an ideal means to build on strength and understand weaknesses.

If depression is severe, seek immediate medical help.

DIABETES

Diabetes has reached epidemic proportions in the West and is indirectly responsible for one in every eight deaths in the United States and one in every three cases of blindness. It is undoubtedly one of the most insidious diseases of our civilization. Studies of various populations prove that the instance of diabetes rises directly in relation to the consumption of sugar and refined carbohydrates. Eighty per cent of all diabetics have, at some time in the past, been obese. Stress and adrenal exhaustion play a part in diabetes, as do liver damage or toxicity and spinal lesions in the middle of the thoracic area. These should be checked out routinely.

Blood sugar levels react differently for different people in response to the same food, so allergies must be taken into account as one of the factors in diabetes.

The basic problem with diabetes is that the level of glucose in the blood is higher than normal while at the same time it is low inside the cells. This is bought about by the progressive inability of the pancreas to secrete the hormone insulin on demand. Using natural methods to help diabetes has proved successful but much depends on the severity of the case in question and the length of insulin dependency. On several occasions I have managed to wean diabetics who have been on insulin for up to 15 years off their insulin altogether with good herbal and dietary management. Of all diabetics 20% survive on dietary management alone.

Diabetes should be treated under the supervision of a qualified medical herbalist.

DIET

The diet should be a natural one high in fibrous carbohydrates. Any fats eaten should be unsaturated or vegetable. Red meat is forbidden and chicken and fish may be taken only twice a week. Rely instead on vegetarian protein, such as soya. Fresh fruits are permissible in moderation, although fresh fruit juice is not and all fruit must be eaten with a little protein to slow its digestion. Vegetables that are particularly recommended include Jerusalem artichokes, Brussels sprouts, cucumbers, green beans, garlic and avocados. Fruits recommended include grapefruits and bananas. All oatmeal products are highly recommended, including oatbran. The diet should be 80% raw. Natural supplements including spirulina, nutritional yeast and wheatgerm are particularly helpful. A potassium broth taken regularly throughout the day will help to restore mineral and electrolyte loss. The pattern of meals should be the same as for hypoglycaemia (see page 179).

Other herbs and foods which are known to help because of their hypoglycaemic action (that is, they lower blood sugar levels) include allspice, barley, bugleweed, burdock, cabbage, carrot, dandelion, ginseng, lettuce, nettles, olive, onion, pawpaw, peas, spinach, sunflower, sweet potato, turnip, string beans (one cup of string bean tea is equal to at least one unit of insulin). The recommended dose of string bean tea is one cup made from fresh string beans morning, noon and evening. Prepare it as a decoction (see page 42).

Bitter herbs like chicory, dandelion, endive, fenugreek, goat's rue and fringe tree bark also help.

In my experience a sudden change of diet together with the introduction of some of these foods in herbal form will reduce insulin need dramatically. Therefore initially insulin needs to be very closely monitored. It is dangerous for a diabetic to stop or even reduce insulin intake without being under the care of a doctor who is well aware of the consequences of uncontrolled diabetes. The formulation I found particularly successful is Bioforce's Diabetisan (for supplier see Resources Directory).

OTHER AIDS

- Take a very hot shower on rising, directing the shower head as forcefully as you can over the pancreas.
- Apply a castor oil poultice to the pancreas (located behind the stomach) daily as hot as possible.
- Use dry skin brushing twice a day, followed by alternate hot and cold showers, to improve the metabolism and circulation.
- Hard outdoor exercise such as jogging, swimming or digging the garden will actually reduce the need for insulin.
- Diabetes is more prevalent in soft-water areas so drink lots of mineralized water which contains chromium and other trace elements. Absorption of chromium from chromic chloride is extremely poor, less than 1%. In order for chromium to be biologically active it must be combined with nicotinic acid (vitamin B_3) and several amino acids. This composite compound, called the Glucose

Tolerance Factor (GTF), binds with insulin to improve the utilization of insulin by cells 10 times. Chromium GTF is found in high concentrations in nutritional yeast (its GTF activity is higher than any other food).

- Fasting is inadvisable for diabetics; however, they should avoid all mental and nervous stresses and strains. Such strains exhaust the adrenal glands and considerably slow any healing.

DIARRHOEA

This is caused by a substance irritating the colon so badly that peristalsis goes into overdrive in an attempt to expel it. Occasionally the build-up of old faeces trapped in the colon becomes so large that this itself induces a state of continuous rapid peristalsis, which results in chronic diarrhoea. In other words, odd though it may sound, severe constipation can actually manifest as diarrhoea. It may therefore be helpful to describe what the ideal bowel movement is, especially in view of the fact that many people are embarrassed about actually inspecting their bowel movements.

THE IDEAL BOWEL MOVEMENT

- The faeces should be buoyant when passed; if they sink they are heavy with mucus.
- They should emerge easily, all in one piece and almost immediately you sit down on the toilet. As they float they should begin to break up. It it takes you more than a few minutes to complete a bowel movement you are constipated.
- Faeces should be lightish brown in colour. If their colouring resembles that of the food you have been eating (for example greenish-brown after lots of green vegetables), you have not digested the food properly. If they look yellow or chalky you have a problem with bile secretion or the production of digestive enzymes.
- They should not smell foul, though they will have a slight odour. If you go on a fruit fast for a week and the resulting faeces smell only of the fruit you have eaten, you can be confident that you have a clean colon.
- They should be four-fifths as bulky as the food you have ingested and they should not be compacted.
- They should emerge unaccompanied by foaming, gurgling, flatulence and general orchestration.

It is quite normal to have a bowel movement three times daily as long as the stool is formed and does not contain undigested food particles. Chronic or recurrent diarrhoea may be the result of long-term use of antibiotics and its after-effects, intestinal parasites, food intolerance, digestive-enzyme deficiency, candidiasis, food poisoning, heavy metal poisoning, prolonged stress, severe B complex deficiencies or excessive vitamin C or zinc, pancreatic or adrenal malfunction, anaemia or colitis.

ACUTE DIARRHOEA

Fast on purified water with a squeeze of fresh lemon juice in it and take a warm camomile enema unless colitis is suspected. If colitis is suspected, omit the enema. Take one teaspoon three to five times daily of the Intestinal Corrective No. 3.

Alternatively, take two capsules of bioacidophilus every half hour (for supplier see Resources Directory). Once the diarrhoea stops eat well-ripened mashed bananas with soya yogurt for a further day and then gently wean yourself back on to a normal healthy diet.

If the diarrhoea lasts longer than two to three days it might be the result of colitis or coeliac disease so seek further professional medical help.

INTESTINAL CORRECTIVE NO. 3

Equal parts of:
Apple fruit pectin
pharmaceutical grade bentonite clay
psyllium seed and husks
fenugreek seed
slippery elm inner bark
sycamore or white willow charcoal.

INFANTILE DIARRHOEA

This can be extremely serious if it doesn't clear up within 24 hours. If this is the case, seek immediate urgent medical attention.

Causes of diarrhoea in babies may include overfeeding, a poor natural diet if the mother is breastfeeding, teething, a bacterial or viral infection or intestinal parasites like giardia, threadworms, ascaria and amoeba which are now endemic in the UK. One in five British schoolchildren is infected with parasitic threadworm. Feed the baby on purified water, home-made barley water and home-made potassium broth with plenty of garlic in it. Also give sips of raspberry leaf infusion with a pinch of cinnamon in each cup.

If in doubt seek immediate professional help. Parasitic diarrhoea requires the help of a medical herbalist familiar with such matters.

BARLEY WATER

Pour 1.5 pts (850 ml) of water over 1 oz (30 g) whole barley grains and boil until the quantity is reduced to half. Add the zest and rind of a lemon for flavour although babies don't seem to mind taking it as it is. Strain and drink at room temperature.

POTASSIUM BROTH

It is important to use organic vegetables to make potassium broth. You do not want to consume any toxic insecticides or chemical fertilizers while you are on a cleansing and detoxification programme.

Drink 1 pt (575 ml) or more daily, warmed. Store strained excess in the fridge for up to two days in a glass container and reheat as needed.

Fill one-quarter of a large pot with thickly cut potato peelings, then add equal amounts of carrot peelings and whole chopped beetroot, chopped onions and garlic, and celery and greens. Add hot chili peppers to taste. Add enough water to cover the vegetables and simmer on very low heat for 1–2 hours.

Strain the liquid and drink only the broth. Put the vegetables on the compost. Make only enough for two days, then start a fresh broth.

TRAVELLER'S DIARRHOEA

Certain famous allopathic anti-diarrhoea remedies are now banned in Japan and Sweden after they have been found to cause severe eye and nerve damage. A much safer way to prevent diarrhoea when travelling abroad is to take two tablets of betaine hydrochloride after each meal (for suppliers see Resources Directory). Hydrochloric acid effectively kills any malign bacteria in the stomach and prevents infection. Alternatively, eating raw garlic daily is an excellent preventative and to a lesser extent undiluted lemon or lime juice taken on an empty stomach has an antiseptic sterilizing effect.

DIVERTICULITIS

Nearly 30% of people beyond middle age in the Western world suffer from diverticular disease and Merck's manual categorically states that 100% of people over the age of 65 suffer from it. In under-developed countries it is almost unknown. It occurs where there is a weakness in the wall of the colon which can develop into a pouch called a diverticulum. The pouches are most commonly found in the sigmoid colon – that is, the last section of the colon before it reaches the rectum. They become filled with bacteria and consume a large amount of B vitamins; blood loss may also occur. Once inflamed any fibrous indigestible material like seeds or skins from fruit can cause intense pain in the lower abdomen (often mistaken for appendicitis) occasionally accompanied by nausea, vomiting and a distended abdomen. Constipation and diarrhoea may alternate.

The solution is high-fibre diet, but where there is inflammation the initial approach must be a low-fibre one until the inflammation has subsided. Fast on a single fruit or vegetable juice until all the painful symptoms have decreased consistently. Then gently begin to add baked or steamed root vegetables, well-ripened mashed bananas, and pawpaw. Move on to puréed stewed fruit and then cautiously on to grated raw foods avoiding pips and skins. Then introduce whole grains, which must be well chewed, and steamed fish. This whole process generally takes between six and eight weeks. Three cups of slippery elm gruel daily will help to heal the intestinal walls. Take the Intestinal Corrective No. 3 formulation (see page 152). Begin with one heaped teaspoon in 6 fl oz (175 ml) of juice with each meal and increase to five heaped teaspoons over the course of a day, if necessary. If pain is acute, apply a castor oil compress to the abdomen leaving it on for up to four hours, and also take hot and cold sitz-baths daily.

Once the diet has been adjusted go on to the diet recommended for constipation following through Intestinal Corrective Formula No. 1 (page 143). Initially you may find the high-fibre approach causes flatulence and some pain but the body, properly nurtured, will soon settle down. Remember cellulose actively encourages friendly bacterial development, which in turn produces several of the B complex vitamins in the intestines. Raw sprouted alfalfa is especially helpful for deodorizing the diverticulum.

DIZZINESS SEE MÉNIÈRE'S DISEASE
DUODENAL ULCER

Ulcers are the result of gastric over-acidity and, in the under-35s, executive stress plays a large part in them, but recent research has pinned the main blame on an infection from bacteria.

Sometimes known as gastric ulcers, these can be caused by a variety of factors including delayed gastric emptying, over-secretion of hydrochloric acid, deranged stomach lining and a washback of bile from the duodenum. Ulcers are certainly exacerbated by drugs, particularly aspirin, steroids, non-steroid anti-inflammatory drugs (NSAIDs), cigarettes, alcohol, tea, coffee, vinegar, spices and, of course, prolonged stress. Stomach ulcers are almost unknown in primitive societies which means that an unrefined diet must surely play a large part in their prevention. Only men used to suffer from ulcers but they are becoming more apparent as one of the penalties hard-working female executives are paying for their stressful jobs.

The new research into *H. pylori* has unearthed the presence of an organism (*Helicobacter pylori*) causes the majority of cases of ulcer: 80% of stomach ulcers and 98% of duodenal ulcers. Research implicating it in causing ulcers is still very new, but it has been suggested that the inflammation caused by the organism appears to interfere with the inhibitory mechanism of acid secretion in the stomach, causing an over-production of acids. *H. pylori* is associated with a two- to six-fold increase of gastric cancer. In the Western world the infection occurs in about one-quarter of symptom-free adults increasing to about 50% by the time the person reaches their middle years. It is caught from close contact which is one reason why ulcers appear to run in families.

ALLOPATHIC TREATMENT

Enlightened doctors are beginning to treat H. *pylori* with a potent cocktail of chemicals including amoxycillin (an antibiotic), metronidazole (an anti-proto-zoal) and bismuth (an anti-ulcer preparation). Any of these used singularly is only about 30% effective, but there are problems with this chemical arsenal; you can expect to suffer:

- profound and debilitating diarrhoea
- nausea
- vomiting
- drowsiness
- headaches
- dizziness and vertigo
- irritability
- depression
- insomnia
- confusion
- hives
- fever
- cystitis.

In addition, you may face the side effects associated with antibiotics and those associated with bismuth, including the possibility of serious ulceration, stomatitis or kidney failure.

HERBAL HELP

A paste made from equal parts of goldenseal and slippery elm together with grapefruit seed extract has a broad range of anti-bacterial activity, including H. *pylori* and campylobacter. It is also anti-fungal and anti-parasitic and, most pleasing of all, it is not toxic and so has no side effects. It is available from Biocare and Higher Nature (see Resources Directory).

Plenty of raw, fresh garlic juiced in the following drinks will underline its action. Raw, freshly pressed cabbage or potato juice is helpful. Juiced separately or in equal proportions and mixed together the final result is rather unpalatable, so mix half and half with celery or carrot juice. Aim to drink four or five glasses daily and adhere closely to the food-combining rules, as well as a vegan diet. I have helped patients to heal gastric ulcers within four to five weeks if all these instructions are carefully followed. The following powdered herbs mixed singly or in equal parts into vegetable juice also help: comfrey, liquorice, peppermint, marshmallow, slippery elm.

Dr Christopher, one of the best-known herbalists in America, had great success using cayenne pepper to heal stomach ulcers. He prescribed one heaped teaspoonful three times a day in water.

Seek the advice of a qualified medical herbalist.

EARACHE

Ears are very delicate, sensitive, complex organs and can easily be permanently damaged by neglect or inappropriate treatment. If in doubt, consult a qualified medical herbalist. Ear infections are common and are often the result of blocked Eustachian tubes which allow mucus to gather within the ear, an ideal medium for bacterial proliferation. Babies are particularly susceptible to earache and many do have an ear infection with almost every viral or bacterial upper respiratory infection. The problem is they can't tell you what is wrong but can only scratch at their ears or pull them or, more likely, yell. Babies are particularly sensitive to secondhand smoke which can often create earaches, as can allergies to specific foods, particularly milk and wheat. Never nurse a baby while lying down as this position encourages milk to gather at the back of the throat instead of being digested naturally downward.

Judging by the number of grommets inserted into the ears of my young patients, chronic ear infection is on the increase. Chronically enlarged adenoids are an indication of a deeper disorder and it is in correcting the conditions that lead to their enlargement that a true cure may be found and grommets avoided (see Tonsillitis). A mucus-free diet is extremely helpful with the addition of mucus-cleansing foods such as garlic and onions, as well as plenty of carrot juice.

The people most affected by external ear infections tend to produce a lot of heavy ear wax which is partly related to diet. To reverse the tendency to produce excessive ear wax cut out saturated fats and take 1,500 mg flax seed or evening primrose oil. It is essential to begin treatment for every ear infection right at the beginning of the problem. Tune in to early signs (congestion in the ear, loss of hearing, pressure or slight pain or the inability to clear the ears). If you have an upper respiratory infection adhere to a mucus-cleansing diet immediately and make sure you clear your ears after blowing your nose. If the earache is the result of a chill, apply a raw grated onion poultice over the back and sides of the neck securing it in place with a cotton bandage. Put a few drops of mullein oil into both ears, even if the earache is only in one ear, and plug with cottonwool. Keep the head, neck and the ears warm at all times.

Garlic oil and garlic foot poultices are particularly useful for ear infections if a child will not adhere to a mucus-free diet.

Something particularly good for ear infections is an oil consisting of equal parts of St John's wort, mullein, tea-tree and garlic oil. Hot compresses of camomile applied directly to the ears and neck are especially useful for acute pain. Alternate hot and cold compresses of camomile are better for chronic pain.

ECZEMA

This is characterized by inflamed, itchy red skin eruptions which sometimes contain small bubbles just beneath the skin surface which can break, producing a weeping rash. The term dermatitis – which simply means inflammation of the skin – is almost interchangeable with eczema and even though allopathic medicine tends to grace it with different terms the differences are not important as far as a holistic approach is concerned.

Contact eczema or dermatitis which tends to be very common in adults involves avoiding the factor which triggers it off, whether that is a chemical, perfume, plant, metal or an item of clothing.

Nutritionally, people with eczema are much more likely to have a zinc deficiency coupled with a disturbance to the metabolism of essential fatty acids. Many of them are allergic to food such as dairy products, eggs, fish, food additives and sugar. If eczema started just after the child was weaned, a mother needs to look back carefully at recently introduced foods. Eczema in a breastfed baby is rare and may be the result of something that the mother is eating. This needs investigation.

An iridology test is particularly useful for determining whether the liver, kidneys or nervous system have been disrupted. In my experience the most common causes of eczema – and indeed all other skin diseases – are found in faulty metabolism, poor elimination of toxic wastes and nutritional deficiencies. Juice fasting will often reap a very marked improvement. There will generally be a worsening of the condition during a fast as the result of an increased elimination of waste matter through the skin but as fasting continues the improvement will become obvious very quickly.

MESSEGUE'S FORMULA FOR ECZEMA SUFFERERS

Maurice Messegue, a well-known French herbalist, claimed a 98% success rate with the following treatment.

First boil up 1 quart (1.1 litre) of water in a glass or enamel saucepan (never use aluminium or copper) then let it cool down until it is lukewarm. Add to this a handful of each of the following herbs (use fresh if possible, dried if fresh are out of season):
artichoke leaves
elecampane (leaves or flowers)
celandine (leaves)
chicory (tips and roots)
broom (flowers)
lavender (flowers)
nettle leaves

Allow the mixture to soak in a covered vessel for five hours and then strain and pour into clean sterilized bottles for storage in the fridge. The extract will last for up to eight days before a new one needs to be brewed.

The extract is then used for an eight-minute foot bath each morning before breakfast and each evening before dinner. To make the bath, boil up 2 quarts of water (2.25 litres) and let it stand for five minutes, add 10 fl oz (300 ml) of the plant extract to the water and immerse the feet or hands into the water as hot as you

*can tolerate. The bath preparation can be kept and warmed for the next bath but do
not add boiling water or any other water.*

Messegue's recipe is complex but works extremely well; for children's eczema,
however, I have found heartsease helpful. Give the tincture according to the age
of the child three times a day in juice. Adult eczema often responds well to blood-
cleansing herbs and nervines. I have found eczema responds well to a correction of
fatty-acid deficiency. Such a deficiency can cause skin rashes resembling eczema
or psoriasis. If this is the case reduce saturated fat and increase unsaturated fat
intake while avoiding commercially transformed or overheated unsaturated fats
such as margarine or deep-fried foods which are overloaded with harmful transfatty acids known to interfere with normal essential fatty-acid metabolism. Also
add to the diet oils which are particularly high in gamma-linoleic acid and linoleic
acid such as flax seed, sunflower, safflower and evening primrose oil. The only
other dietary source of this is human breast milk, which protects against infantile
eczema.

EMPHYSEMA

Emphysema may result from inhaling industrial pollution, radioactive fallout,
and cigarette smoking. Improvement with herbal treatment is possible
although it must be recognized that some parts of the lungs may remain
scarred for life. Because this disease is so serious, it needs very careful
supervision and management and therefore you are advised to seek the help
of a medical herbalist.

Follow a general good diet. All exercise should be gentle and progressive and
carried out in an atmosphere where the mucous membranes of the lungs will not
dry out, so swimming in water which is cleaned by ozone is ideal. Spinal
manipulation may be helpful. Activities such as singing, whistling or playing a
musical instrument which involves forceful breathing out helps to develop lung
efficiency. (I was once consulted by a miner from South Wales who helped his
emphysema to an extraordinary degree by practising pranayama yogic breathing
and hatha yoga on a twice daily basis.)

**Emphysema is a serious condition and should only be treated by a
qualified practitioner**.

ENDOMETRIOSIS

This is the result of the tissue lining the womb becoming misplaced and adhering
to other parts of the body, commonly the ovaries, Fallopian tubes and peritoneum,
although deposits have been found all over the body including the lungs and the
eyes. These deposits behave as if they were womb lining and bleed during every

menstrual period. The bleeding causes inflammation and adhesions can form which can make organs stick to one another.

This is the second most common gynaecological problem, requiring hospital treatment, and researchers are still investigating its causes. There is now a emerging a close link between dioxin (toxic chemical) levels in the body and the severity and incidence of endometriosis. This being the case, women may prefer not to use sanitary towels or tampons but find alternatives such as natural sponges or washable cotton sanitary towels (for suppliers see Resources Directory). As dioxins are airborne and can fall on grass and plants eaten by farmed animals it is also essential to cut out all dairy produce from the diet.

Endometriosis commonly occurs in women between the ages of 30 and 45; pregnancy protects a woman from endometriosis (conventional treatment is to use the contraceptive pill to suppress ovulation and menstruation) which often begins to disappear after the menopause. This may be because endometriosis may be hormonally linked to an over-production of oestrogen, which ceases after the menopause. As a result, HRT has been shown to reactivate symptoms by releasing oestrogen into the bloodstream of post-menopausal women. Current drug therapy for endometriosis aims to suppress ovulation, by inducing a state similar to pregnancy or the menopause. Danazol, one of the most commonly used drugs for endometriosis, and another drug, Gestrinone, induce a post-menopausal state. These are androgens similar to male reproductive hormones. Their side effects include non-reversible hairiness and voice changes as well as greasy skin and acne. Surgeons can remove the lining of the womb to stop heavy bleeding using a variety of techniques, including laser, but this is a risky procedure. Hysterectomy is an option once childbearing is complete.

I have had considerable success working with women with endometriosis but persistence and discipline are necessary. I use a treatment for fibroids. If there is pain I use a nervine sedative and I always advise hot and cold sitz-baths morning and evening with 10 drops of cypress oil added to the water.

Although the contraceptive pill unhibits ovulation, it may not protect against endometriosis and in some cases has actually been implicated in causing the condition.

ENURESIS

By the age of three and a half 75% of all children in the Western world at least have acquired bladder control both day and night; by the age of five the figure is 90%. Don't worry about bed wetting, unless it happens frequently after the age of six or seven, but attend to any anxiety in the child.

Inflammation of the bladder is rare among children. Common symptoms include pain and burning on urination, cloudy, sour smelling, or bloody urination, backache, chills and high fevers. Make sure your child is not wearing clothes washed by bleaches and detergents next to the skin and avoid fabric coloured by chemical dyes in their underwear. Do not let them wash with soap, particularly around the genital area. Running water will do just as well. Give them a cup of cranberry juice, preferably unsweetened, morning and evening with two drops of tea-tree oil added to each cup, and encourage them to drink plenty of potassium broth. If they complain of soreness use a warm compress of fennel oil, 10 drops diluted in enough water to moisten the compress, over the bladder and wrap them up well, keeping the rest of the body warm.

In only 3% of children with enuresis is there an organic cause to the condition, although the incidence of organic causes becomes more frequent in the older groups; in 75% of all adolescents who suffer enuresis there is an organic cause. Those include chronic infection, a stricture of the urethra, and ectopic urethral insertion into the bladder or some other kind of obstruction. Hypoglycaemia can cause enuresis because hypoglycaemics tend to enter a deep sleep which does not allow the part of the brain responsible for social awareness to receive the signal of a full bladder. Occasionally food – particularly dairy – allergy is to blame. It is worth considering spinal lesions which may disrupt the normal flow of circulation to the bladder. An iridology test will show them clearly and referral to an osteopath is necessary in these cases. Spinal lesions are much more common than was once supposed and can be caused by birth trauma or any one of the more serious falls that toddlers seem to suffer so frequently. Such lesions may disrupt the normal flow of both nerve impulses and circulation to the bladder.

Finally, psychological causes of enuresis are now well acknowledged. It is not uncommon for an older child to develop enuresis when a second child arrives as a way to gain attention or even a desire to return to an earlier stage of development with more parental care. Emotions attached to enuresis include anxiety, fear, resentment or even the desire to get even with the parent in question. Punishment will not make the situation better and it is vital that the child be made to feel secure understands this is not a 'problem'. Measure the child's volume capacity during the course of the day. If you can collect between 8 and 10 fl oz (250 and 300 ml) at a time, the problem is not one of a small bladder.

To treat, limit (but do not bar) fluids in the last couple of hours before bed and make sure the bladder is fully emptied before going to bed. If the child is really thirsty offer a juicy piece of fruit, rather than a drink, but sending a child to bed longing for a drink solves nothing and may, in fact, make matters worse. There should be no salt in the diet. Massage the kidneys daily with warm olive oil and encourage the child to sleep on his or her side, rather than the back. Give three cups of equal parts of parsley and corn tassel tea daily: this won't irritate tender tummies or the urinary tract.

Foot baths of corn tassel also help (for correct administration see page 49). Cold sitz-baths are particularly helpful if the child can be persuaded to take them for five minutes morning and evening.

Depending on the age of the child Kegel exercises may be helpful because they teach the child to contract the appropriate muscles to the bladder.

EPILEPSY

Many cases of epilepsy are misdiagnosed so, before treating it, make sure that you do have a correct diagnosis particularly as the drugs used for epilepsy are extremely strong and have many side effects. When planning a diet for an epileptic ensure that all possible allergens are eliminated. I have found intolerances to mercury fillings in several of my epileptic patients. Diet must be adequate in magnesium-rich foods supplemented with magnesium supplements as magnesium deficiency has been shown to be involved in epilepsy. The diet should also be a hypoglycaemic one as low blood sugar can also be involved in epilepsy (see the diet for hypoglycaemia on page 177). The best natural sources of magnesium are nuts, seeds, soya beans and green leafy vegetables. If vegetables are cooked, the cooking water should be consumed. Epileptics, while keeping mentally active and avoiding all sorts of mental or physical stresses, should take care not to get extremely excited, angry or full of fear or hatred, which often provokes attacks. Plenty of rest during menstruation, pregnancy and the menopause are required by epileptics because these times often provoke seizures. A warm dry climate is preferable: seizures seem to increase in frequency during cold winters and rainstorms with high humidity. Physical activity out in clean fresh air is particularly advisable as it will oxygenate the brain cells. Epsom salt baths taken twice weekly are beneficial (see page 47).

DR CHRISTOPHER'S TINCTURE

Dr Christopher advised the following tincture with which he had over many years in practice a great deal of success. This will feed and calm the nervous system and reduce hyperactivity.
Equal parts of:
black cohosh
lady's slipper
skullcap
lobelia (available only from a qualified medical herbalist)
vervain.

Take 30 drops four times a day and also rub it into the back of the neck to influence the medulla regulatory centre and calm breathing and basic bodily functions. Ensure that all eliminative channels are kept working well.

Epilepsy should be treated by a qualified medical herbalist.

FATIGUE

Prolonged stress not only batters our nervous system but can also do insidious damage to our glandular system, particularly to the adrenal glands. There are two main benefits of the stable functioning of adrenal hormones: firstly, abundant energy and secondly, a super-charged immune system able to fight off disease quickly, completely and with the minimum of fuss.

If you are so tired you simply can't be bothered about anything and life is just too short even to try, your adrenalin is low. The danger here is not only to your personality but to your ability to fight off disease quickly and completely. People often say to me, 'I wish I had your energy to do all the things you do,' and my question is: 'So, what is stopping you? Fear? Hopelessness? Despair? Laziness? Lack of self-esteem? Alcohol? Drugs? Smoking? Lack of exercise?'

There is no one natural remedy for restoring sexual drive. Certainly good nutrition helps, particularly magnesium and zinc, but an abundance of adrenal hormone will also stimulate the ovaries into action.

ADRENAL TONIC

The following formulation is designed to restore hormonal function, support the adrenal glands, regulate blood sugar and increase the body's resistance to disease, so helping counteract stress. It is also good for jetlag if taken a week before the flight and a week after.
Two parts of:
Siberian ginseng
One part of:
echinacea
wild oats
bladderwrack
gotu kola.
This should be made as a tincture and 15 drops taken four or five times a day.

CHRONIC EXHAUSTION

The following formulation will help the adrenal glands by nourishing and supporting them in the long term. This is useful when stress has been chronic.
One part of:
ginger
cayenne pepper
dandelion
milk thistle
Half a part of:
damiana
lavender
St John's wort.

Take three size 0 capsules morning and evening.

FEVER SEE CHILDHOOD DISEASES

FIRST AID

Every household should have a well-stocked first-aid cabinet at the ready in case of an emergency. Accidents are the most common cause of death in children between the ages of one and 14. Yet most serious accidents can easily be prevented. People, particularly children, are more likely to have accidents when they are sick, tired, cranky, excited, distracted, unhappy, jealous or worried. Children are also prone to particular accidents: some fall, some pinch their fingers, some get burned, some ingest poisons. A study carried out on poisoning shows that 25% of all children who ingest poisons will have a second episode of ingestion within a year. The more parents understand their children's tendencies the more effectively they can safety-proof their environment and work to educate their child.

This section is not designed to qualify anyone in first aid and it does not have detailed instructions for bandaging, splinting, suturing or setting broken bones. All these can be learned at a first-aid class and everyone is urged to attend at least one. Most people are terrified at the mere thought of an accident and wouldn't know what to do if one occurred. Learning the most effective way to respond to any accident will help to relieve much of this terror; attendance at a first-aid course is the first step to doing this.

There are two accident situations in which prompt action is essential:

- When a person has stopped breathing due to choking, electric shock or drowning. If breathing has stopped resuscitation should begin within minutes and such resuscitation is taught at first-aid classes.
- When a person is bleeding severely due to a large cut or puncture wound. If someone is bleeding severely a firm pressure should be applied directly. Only very serious bleeding from a major artery requires the use of a tourniquet and this is best applied by somebody properly trained in first aid: improper use can actually result in blood vessel and nerve damage.

Most accidents are not serious and they rarely are true emergencies in the sense that it is important to act or get help immediately. In nearly every accident you will have enough time to comfort the victim and calm them down (as well as calming yourself, of course), before you even evaluate the extent of the injury. Calming the 'patient' is the first important step in treating most scrapes, stings, bites, cuts, burns, bumps and falls. But there may be situations where you are far away from home, for example, when there simply isn't the time or the facility to look up medical treatment and basic knowledge beforehand can be very useful. You are therefore advised to read the following sections thoroughly and memorize anything you feel may be important: bites, burns (including sunburn), childhood diseases, frostbite, insect bites and stings, minor cuts and bruises, miscarriage, nosebleeds, poisoning, septicaemia, shock, sprains, teething, toothache, travel sickness, wounds.

ESSENTIAL HERBAL PREPARATION FOR A FIRST-AID CABINET

- The following seeds in their whole form: caraway, dill, fennel.
- A small supply of each of the following herbs: cayenne, chaparral, false unicorn, ginger, lobelia (obtainable only on prescription from a qualified medical herbalist), slippery elm.
- The following tinctures: arnica, cayenne, echinacea, goldenseal, lobelia, plantain.
- The most important essential oils are: lavender, rosemary, thyme.
- Tea-tree oil is also useful as is deep heat oil and trauma oil (for suppliers see Resources Directory).
- Ensure you have a bottle of Dr Bach's Rescue Remedy (see Resources Directory) as well as some vitamin E oil in capsule form, a small jar of organic runny honey, several garlic cloves, comfrey ointment and marigold cream.
- A bottle of witch hazel is always useful for sprains, and elderflower, peppermint and yarrow herbs should be kept at the ready for fevers.

FLATULENCE SEE GASTRITIS
FRIGIDITY SEE IMPOTENCE
FROSTBITE

Rapidly warm up the area by taking a warm bath of about 110°F (43°C). Take care not to overdo the heat or you will burn the frozen skin. Pat dry gently: do not rub. Administer Dr Bach's Rescue Remedy internally and externally (see Resources Directory) if necessary every 15 minutes and seek immediate medical help. Generally there are few complications but if improperly handled the condition may lead to gangrene so don't attempt to treat this by yourself.

GALL STONES

If the bile duct from the liver is blocked, sudden jaundice may ensue, but gall stones are generally the result of bile stasis so the gall bladder is only partially emptied. This thickened bile combined with a faulty high cholesterol diet may induce cholecystitis (inflammation of the gall bladder) where gall stones get stuck in the neck of the gall bladder causing biliary colic. This is extremely painful, although not generally as painful as kidney stones.

Surgery never helps to correct the cause of gall stones or the disease. It only serves to denude the body of a useful organ.

Over 90% of gall stones are made of cholesterol and the phospholipid concentration in the bile of gall stones patients is lower than normal. Two tablespoons of lecithin granules (see Resources Directory) will help to increase the phospholipid concentration and so work toward dispersing and preventing the formation of gall stones, providing it is coupled with colic acid (a constituent of normal bile).

The pill doubles the chances of gall stones simply because it decreases the vitamin E content in the body so if you wish to continue taking the pill take vitamin E with it: 400 IUs to start with (unless there is a history of rheumatic fever in the family) and thereafter increase to 1000IUs; in this case vitamin E is contraindicated as it may raise the blood pressure and burden the heart.

Diet should be vegetarian or, better still, vegan with an emphasis on vegetable juices and raw or lightly cooked vegetables together with plenty of fresh pears, grapes, apples and grapefruit (which are particularly cleansing fruits for the gall bladder) and a complete abstinence from meat and saturated or denatured fats such as margarine.

In acute attacks fast on diluted grape juice only and apply cold castor oil compresses to the liver. Calcareous stones, however, cannot be removed by this method (for their removal see page 83).

GASTRITIS

Indigestion, heartburn and gastritis are symptoms of abnormal digestion rather than diseases in themselves. Allopathically they are normally treated with antacids and their cause is seldom tackled. Used on a regular basis such antacids upset the body's acid–alkaline balance creating alkalosis. Sustained alkalosis, with a substantial intake of calcium by way of milk or calcium-coating antacids, creates milk-alkali syndrome causing irreversible kidney damage.

The easiest way to cope with such digestive disorders is to follow the food-combining rules.

- Do not combine protein with starch.
- Eat fruits separately, and in isolation.
- Take no liquids with meals except for herbal teas and vegetable juices. A glass of wine or two of excellent quality is permissible occasionally.

Avoid excessively large meals and chew really well so that plenty of ptyalin, the digestive enzyme salivary amylase, is mixed with carbohydrate in the mouth. Not only does thorough chewing stimulate salivary amylase secretions so breaking down food into smaller particles for more complete exposure for enzymic digestion, but it also stimulates the secretion of digestive enzymes in the stomach, pancreas and small intestine so facilitating digestion further. Of course you need to chew really well to break down indigestible cellulose found in all vegetables to expose their innerfood substances to digestive juices.

Excessively hot or cold foods irritate the delicate stomach lining.

Never, never, eat while stressed.

Do not eat when sick. All animals (it seems with the exception of human beings) fast when they are ill.

Make sure that you haven't any food allergies and, if these are suspected, have them tested.

Do not eat cooked food late at night.

Do not cook with copper or aluminium.

Avoid gastric irritants including spices, sugar, coffee, fizzy drinks and alcohol, and especially avoid salt which is the most common irritant to the stomach. It causes acidity and irritates the stomach's delicate mucous membranes.

If you suspect digestive enzyme deficiency – and it is possible to be tested for this (see Resources Directory) – take digestive enzymes. Those made from pawpaw and pineapple are excellent. Hydrochloric acid deficiency is a common problem especially in the over-40s causing poor protein assimilation and chronic malabsorption of many vitamins and minerals.

We tend to think that heartburn is the result of hyperacidity whereas in fact it is the result of hypoacidity, which is why antacids make the condition worse. Milk will exacerbate the condition since it takes so much hydrochloric acid to acidify milk. Note, hydrochloric acid deficiency can also cause hypothyroidism, allergies, asthma, rheumatoid arthritis, anaemia, diabetes, systemic candidiasis, chronic hepatitis, parasitic invasion, eczema and vitiligo. With this in mind, it is well worth checking for this deficiency.

Finally, spinal lesions over the thoracic area can distort the nerve and blood supply to the stomach and other digestive organs, so it is worth getting checked by an osteopath or chiropractor.

For acute or chronic indigestion fast on apple or carrot juice, slippery elm gruel and water with a squeeze of lemon. Continue with the fast until the condition has completely subsided and then go on a mono-diet regime of either carrots, apples or brown rice for at least 24 hours, or until the problem has cleared.

Always begin therapy with fast and dietary changes before resorting to herbal medicine. Often a simple change in regime is enough to cure the problem permanently.

GINGIVITIS

This is an extremely common bacterial infection of the outermost tissues of the gums, caused by lack of oral hygiene and a poor diet.

Seek the advice of your dentist urgently.

The following remedies are helpful.

- Switch to a non-fluoridated toothpaste containing echinacea or myrrh.
- Use a mouth rinse of equal parts of echinacea and myrrh several times a day.
- Massage oil of eucalyptus into the gum just before bed. It tastes terrible but it is very effective. Rinse out the next morning with a mouth wash.
- Ensure the diet has an adequate quantity of vitamins A, D and C and avoid refined carbohydrates and processed foods.

Many people have no idea how to clean their teeth properly. You should dislodge food particles between the teeth which can cause plaque formation with waxed dental floss (a dental hygienist will show you how to use this correctly) and then use a soft toothbrush with rounded bristles spreading it with a little of the toothpaste recommended above. The brush should then be held at an angle of 45° to the teeth, and the teeth should be gently scrubbed following this angle. Having rinsed the mouth give the gums a good massage using the fingertips in a small rotary movement. Alternatively use an electric toothbrush, but make sure it is a soft one and massage the gums after cleaning the teeth.

GLANDULAR FEVER SEE MONONUCLEOSIS
GLAUCOMA SEE CATARACTS AND GLAUCOMA
GOITRE

This is an enlargement of the thyroid gland characterized by a swelling around the front of the neck and is generally due to iodine deficiency. Watercress and seaweed are both rich sources of iodine. But certain foods actually inhibit the utilization of iodine. They include peanuts, soya flour, Brussels sprouts, cauliflower, cabbage, kale, broccoli, turnips and kohl rabi. Obviously these should be avoided in the instance of a goitre; vitamin E deficiency reduces iodine absorption by 95%.

In some countries synthetic iodine is added to salt in the belief that this will solve the problem. However, natural sources of iodine are needed. In those people whose thyroid secretion is already excessive, iodine salt can lead to palpitations or Basedow's disease (exophthalmic goitre). In any case, salt is harmful in general in the diet.

A very effective Swiss remedy is cabbage and clay poultices prepared with oak bark decoction and applied alternately to the front of the neck. Use one warm poultice followed by the other once it has cooled down.

Specific foods which are helpful include bladderwrack, dulse, kelp, garlic, nutritional yeast, watercress, unsalted seafood, egg yolks and mushrooms, as well as Superfood (see page 18). A remedy that I have used with particular success is nasturtium, available from Bioforce (see Resources Directory).

Seek the advice of a qualified medical herbalist.

GOUT

Gout is caused by the precipitation of insoluble crystals of uric acid into the joints which then become red, swollen and painful. It can be healed by various dietary changes including losing weight, if you are overweight, stopping alcohol completely and following a strict low uric acid and low purine diet which means avoiding all meat (particularly organ meats), eggs, fish and dairy produce – in other words becoming a vegan. The only wheat to be taken should be in sprouted form. Foods high in potassium are protective against gout so potassium broth is indicated (see page 31). Red sour cherries and strawberries are of specific value in gout. Cherries have a remarkable ability to alkalize the system and neutralize uric acid. When they are in season it is advisable to do a three- to four-day fast on them. You may notice, if you try this, a considerable worsening of the condition in the early stages of fasting. This is simply the uric acid, dissolved by the juices from the fruit, being thrown into the bloodstream for elimination and it will clear up if fasting continues faithfully. A series of short three- to four-day fasts is preferable to one long fast and much more comfortable.

I often cheer my gout patients up by telling them that research indicates that a high blood level of uric acid is associated with a high level of intellectual attainment.

Megadoses of Vitamin C assist the loss of uric acid through the kidneys; take up to 4 a day. Drink three cups of the following infusion daily: equal parts of celery, boneset, burdock root, Irish moss, alfalfa. If the pain is particularly bad add half a part of goldenseal and half a part of thuja.

GUM DISEASE

Pyorrhoea is a chronic degenerative disease of the gums where the teeth become loose and the gums spongy. Follow the advice for gingivitis (see page 166) and clean the teeth with the following tooth powder: equal parts of finely powdered bayberry, bistort, orris root and sage. Rinse afterward with a double-strength decoction of bistort. Then surround the gums around the loose teeth with powdered white oak bark and try, if you can, to leave it on all night. If you swallow a bit it doesn't matter. Continue this treatment nightly until the gums have firmed up. Also treat systemically with high doses of vitamin C, stopping just short of diarrhoea, and the following formulation: two parts echinacea, one part blue flag, one part chaparral. Drink one cup of the tea three times a day with meals until the condition has healed but for not longer than six weeks. You also need to seek the advice of your dentist urgently.

HAEMORRHOIDS AND ANAL FISSURE

Haemorrhoids are a very painful condition, and surgery does nothing to prevent a recurrence. It only creates yet more scar tissue. An anal fissure, a split in the anus, is even more painful and because of its location can take a long time to heal.

DIET

Prevent constipation at all costs with a mainly raw diet which is high in fibre, and drink plenty of liquids between meals, but not with meals. Sit on the toilet in the correct way (see page 140). Do daily abdominal strengthening yoga exercises and slant-board exercises.

SLANT-BOARD

A slant-board is simply a strong piece of wood big enough to lie on and positioned so that one end is supported several inches off the floor. Lie with your head at the lower end. Begin with a 3 in (7.5cm) slope but increase this gradually as you get used to it to about 2 ft (60 cm). These exercises help to correct any prolapse in the body whether it be of the uterus, stomach, colon, bladder or anus and they are also useful for other problems including eye, ear and sinus.

....

Caution: A slant-board should not be used by those suffering from hypertension, stomach ulcers, TB, appendicitis, abdominal cancer, those with a tendency to haemorrhage, or during a particularly heavy period.

....

1. With your head at the lower end of the slant-board, breathe in slowly, raise your arms and stretch them above your head, reaching right back so that you touch the floor with the back of your hands behind you. When you get there breathe out and hold for a few seconds. Now breathe in again and and bring your arms back. Rest them by your sides. Repeat this 10 times. On a 3 in (7.5 cm) slant you won't slide off but once you reach 2 ft (60 cm), you'll need to tuck your feet under a wide band of webbing or leather secured round the foot of the board to stay in place.

2. With your arms by your sides, breathe out fully and suck your stomach muscles in so that you feel as if your abdomen is touching your spine. Hold for a few seconds and snap out, at which point you will automatically breathe in again. Relax. Repeat 10 times.

3. Give yourself a stomach massage following the path of the colon from right to left, or if this is initially too strenuous, try rolling a small ball (about the size of a tennis ball) over your lower colon, pressing deeply as you follow its path in a big clockwise circle.

4. Hold onto the side of the board firmly with your hands and slowly bend your knees so that they are resting on your chest. Don't worry if you can't do this fully at first – it will come in time. Now turn your head from side to side (5 times to each side) while holding this position. Then, if you can, lift your head slightly and rotate it, first clockwise, then anti-clockwise (3 times each way), then slowly replace your legs so that they are lying flat on the board.

5. Lift your legs, vertically bending your knees as you do so. Keeping them bent rotate one foot outwards in a circle 10 times, repeat with the other foot, then both together.

6. Cycle with your legs in the air, working up to 25 rotations as a maximum.

7. Now relax and, as you get your breath back, squeeze all the muscles in your face hard, then let them go; as you do so you will feel the tension flooding from your face. As your breathing slows down to normal, feel the tension seeping out of your body. It sometimes helps to imagine it draining out of the top of your head. Rest and relax for a minimum of 5 minutes, letting the recharged blood circulate into your head. Get up slowly.

To relieve pain sit in a hot sitz-bath on folded towels (see page 49) with 10 drops of cypress oil added.

In acute cases where the haemorrhoids have prolapsed use cold sitz-baths with 10 drops of geranium oil added, or insert an ice suppository.

Make a funnel of stiff waxed paper about the size of a tampon evenly rolled so that the hole at the top is the same size as the hole at the bottom and seal it well on the outside with Sellotape. Insert it upright into a piece of plasticine and fill it with water. Freeze. Carefully remove it from the plasticine and unwrap the paper. Insert it into the anus for 1 minute only repeating once more later in the day with a new suppository. Alternatively, apply ice-cold witch hazel on a compress for as long as necessary. In the case of anal fissure inject 4 fl oz (100 ml) cold witch hazel into the anus and retain for 10 minutes.

After every bowel movement sponge with water and pat dry with a flannel. Do not use toilet paper. Having done this apply pilewort ointment internally and externally with the little finger.

To stop the bleeding of piles drink a wine glass of very hot mullein tea sweetened with a little honey 3 times daily.

To shrink haemorrhoids make a decoction of:
2 parts of:
dandelion
stoneroot
1 part of:
agrimony
chicory
Turkey rhubarb
Half a part of:
liquorice
and take a wine glass 3 times daily.

To heal an anal fissure take 10 drops of tormentil tincture in water between meals 3 times daily and insert a suppository of goldenseal powder moulded into a pessary with coconut butter (see below). Do this nightly before going to bed and protect the pants with a press-on sanitary towel as goldenseal stains bright yellow.

TO MAKE A SUPPOSITORY

In a double boiler melt a small piece of coconut butter and, once it is liquid, mix in an equal quantity of finely powdered goldenseal to form a thick paste. Decant the paste on to an oiled wooden board or a marble slab and roll out into sausage pieces the width of your thumb. With a sharp knife carefully cut the sausage into lengths as long as your index finger. Store these on an oiled plate in the refrigerator until they are solid. Each suppository can then be individually wrapped in a little greaseproof paper and stored in a cool place.

HALITOSIS

Halitosis may be the result of a blocked colon or of oral bacteria and I tend to tackle the problem from both angles. First ensure the bowel is clean (see pages 143, 144 and 152), and that the diet includes lots of natural chlorophyll in the form of green tips of freshly sprouted seeds, the juice from wheatgrass (always dilute this 2 fl oz to 8 fl oz (50 ml to 250 ml) of water) and dark green leafy vegetables, and be meticulous about oral hygiene, remembering to floss as well as brush (see the advice for gingivitis on page 166). Chewing a whole clove will sweeten the breath, but only on a temporary basis.

Among those people over 30 who still have their own teeth (one-third do not), three out of four have periodontal disease, that is diseased gums around the teeth. It is the most widespread disease in the world and tends to be relatively painless until well advanced. The first sign is bleeding gums which most people tend to ignore thinking it is the result of over-zealous tooth brushing. Don't be deceived. Go to your dentist immediately and ask to be shown how to both brush and floss your teeth correctly. If left unchecked you will lose your teeth.

HARDENING OF THE ARTERIES: SEE ATHEROSCLEROSIS

HAY FEVER

The treatment of hay fever is often very complex because it is a many-faceted condition. It can be inherited as an allergic predisposition and may initially manifest itself as allergic eczema or asthma as well as food intolerance – it can be triggered by the inhalation of grass pollens or an early intolerance of dairy products, wheat or other foods.

Interestingly, hay fever only seems to have become common over the last 150 years – before this it seems to have been a disease of the educated classes. This raises interesting questions as to its causes. Sugar only began to be taken in large amounts 180 years ago and at that time only the affluent upper classes could afford it. Is there a link here? An intolerance to wheat, which is in the same botanical family as grass, may also be implicated. Take the following steps to alleviate the condition:

- Try to avoid areas with a high pollen count and polluted air – for example, areas in cities where the poisons are often dangerously high. Use an ionizer to control the balance of ions (tiny electrical particles) in the air around you. An ionizer is particularly useful in the bedroom, where you can spend at least 8 of every 24 hours. You can leave the windows open or closed while they are in use; either way they will cope (for suppliers see Resources Directory).
- Because the pollen counts are highest on warm, dry days, it is advisable to stay indoors on such days or ideally go to the seaside and away from fields.
- Stop smoking completely and avoid smoke-filled rooms.
- Use a synthetic duvet and pillows. Feather duvets and pillows tend to attract dust.
- Avoid food additives and foods which commonly cause allergies, such as cow's milk, sucrose, refined carbohydrates, and, in particular, wheat.

Take the following formula. It was used with a great deal of success by Dr Christopher, its originator and the leading herbalist in the USA until his death in 1982. Of course, he also insisted on body purification and correct nutrition too (see Chapters 3 and 4).

DR CHRISTOPHER'S ALLERGY FORMULA

Equal parts of:
burdock root
cayenne
chapparal
ephedra
goldenseal
juniper berries
marshmallow root
parsley root
Half a part of:
lobelia (available only from qualified medical herbalists)

Take two size O capsules three times a day.

The catarrh accumulated during hay fever may be cut by making an infusion of equal parts of ginger and cayenne, adding one crushed clove of garlic and plenty of honey to every cup. Gargle with this and swallow the mixture. Fiery but effective! Take as much of this as often as needed.

This is a difficult condition to treat and as it can result in serious complications if neglected. You are advised to seek the professional help of a medical herbalist if you are not confident about treating it.

HEADACHE

Headaches are evidenced by severe pain in or around the head. Migraines are quite a different matter (see page 201). Stress can rapidly turn painless muscle tension into a headache. If the stress persists, toxins will accumulate in the neck and shoulders and the final result may be osteoarthritis. People – like me – who cup a telephone between the neck and shoulder while writing will exacerbate this problem. It can eased by a few big slow half-head rolls, sitting upright with the shoulders relaxed. (For a half-head roll, do not drop the head back, simply drop the chin forward on the chest.)

Chronic headaches may be the result of:

- liver congestion
- poor circulation

- constipation
- hypoglycaemia
- food intolerance
- sinusitis
- arthritis
- spinal lesions
- anaemia
- the side effects of a lumbar puncture
- meningitis
- brain tumour
- high blood pressure
- eye strain.

....

Some are very serious and others will need only minor correction. Check them all out by consulting a doctor before resorting to self-medication with herbs. A severe headache with vomiting, for example, may be the result of intercerebral haemorrhage which is an emergency.

....

Dandelion and agrimony help if there is liver involvement, peppermint if there is a stomach upset, goldenseal if the headache is bilious, a combination of camomile and peppermint for a sick headache with a nervous stomach, betony if there is vertigo, black cohosh if the headache is of menstrual origin, lavender for pain in the temples (massage one drop of oil into each temple), lemon balm or marjoram for nervous headaches, lime flowers for headaches which begin on the right side and then affect the left side where the head feels dull and congested, pulsatilla for a neurotic headache with menstrual disorders, red clover for headaches accompanied by confusion or a feeling of dread, and vervain for headaches involving muscular tension. All except lavender can be taken as simple herbal teas in infusion or decoction form depending on what part of the plant is being used. Drink a cup as often as needed.

It is important to remember that some herbs, such as valerian and ginseng, can actually cause headaches in some people, and I have had patients react badly to garlic and thyme.

HEART AND CIRCULATORY DISEASE

Coronary heart disease usually expresses itself as angina (that is chest pain on exertion) or a heart attack. Coronary heart disease is the biggest killer in the Western world and affects two out of three people to some degree.

Contrary to popular perception, smoking rather than diet is the major factor associated with any kind of heart disease. It is true that an elevated level of cholesterol in the blood is associated with an increased risk of heart disease but most people simply need to moderate their intake of dietary fats. A fanatical low cholesterol diet is contraindicated (see Atherosclerosis page 115). A diet high in fat and sugars certainly greatly accelerates the risk of heart problems. Don't go on to polyunsaturated margarine (see page 17), which is hydrogenated and comprises as much as 40% transfatty acids which raise cholesterol and inhibit the production of prostaglandins which help lower blood pressure and reduce platelet clumping. Refined cooking oils, those that are not virgin and cold pressed, are unprotected from oxidation and therefore form free radicals which tend to damage artery walls, encouraging atherosclerosis. Free radicals are the result of the failure of an oxidizing atom to add the requisite amount of electrons to complete its formation. This results in an activated molecule which extracts an electron from another donor which consequently becomes altered and may become pathological. Free radicals are directly responsible for the arterial eruptions of atherosclerosis. When using virgin cold-pressed oils add a capsule of vitamin E oil to the bottle and keep it in the fridge when not in use. Use only non-hydrogenated margarines and use these very sparingly.

For those with very severe angina, however, or for people who are at high risk of an heart attack, a vegan diet is ideal. This should also include a liver flush every morning (see page 80). This approach, together with monitored graded exercise, some counselling and learning relaxation techniques, can reduce angina by 91% in less than a month. The flax seed oil in the liver flush will help to prevent platelets sticking to blood vessel walls, as will the ginger and garlic. Vitamin C reduces platelet stickiness in people with coronary heart disease and upward of half a gram needs to be taken daily. Evening primrose oil or borage oil affects prostaglandin metabolism so this also helps to combat platelet stickiness. A combination of hawthorn and motherwort in equal quantities makes a superb heart tonic and antispasmodic. Hawthorn taken faithfully over a period of three months actually helps to strengthen the heart muscle.

In the event of an attack of angina place warm poultices of cider vinegar around the top of the arms and keep changing them as necessary. Alternatively, place a compress of equal parts of hawthorn berries and sage directly over the heart. Leave the compress on for 10 minutes, until cool, and then replace with a very warm one.

Generally I begin my patients on a simple programme of walking on the flat starting with a few minutes with frequent rests and gently building up until they are walking on a slope at a brisk pace for half an hour daily.

....

The following conditions are life-threatening. Seek urgent medical advice and only treat under the supervision of a qualified medical herbalist.

....

HEART ATTACK

There are three main areas in which nutrition is relevant to heart attacks specifically and coronary heart disease generally.

- High cholesterol and triglyceride levels can be controlled by diet and by specific foods within the diet, including evening primrose oil, borage oil, garlic, flax seed and ginger.

- High blood pressure can be controlled by diet and herbal supplementation.
- Platelet stickiness and clotting can be reduced by diet (see above).

The mainstays of treatment in allopathic medicine are intensive care and the use of chemicals to control the heart beat, as well as electric shock to restart the heart. Herbal medicine adopts an altogether gentler approach but is extremely effective. In an emergency situation while waiting for the ambulance/doctor, administer three heaped teaspoons of cayenne in warm water (this to be drunk all at once) and then half a teaspoon every 15 minutes in hot water. Alternatively put 30 drops of tincture of cayenne in a tablespoon of hot water and drink all at once. Then administer 10 drops in a little hot water every 15 minutes. If possible give foot and hand baths of black mustard powder, two handfuls to 1 ¾ pts (1 litre) of water. Rescue Remedy (one of the main Bach Flower Remedies, see Resources Directory) massaged into the wrists, put on the tongue or on the lips is also very helpful for allaying shock and fear. I have even met an enlightened hospital doctor who administered this by intravenous drip.

In a semi-acute situation, nutrition certainly has a substantial part to play not merely by minimizing the effects but hopefully by preventing further heart damage and actively rebuilding the arteries.

PHLEBITIS

When clots form in the veins in the legs, they cause painful localized inflammation, or phlebitis. This is common in pregnant women as the changes in sex hormones during pregnancy cause the blood to clot more rapidly.

Apply external compresses of ice-cold witch-hazel; raw onion rubbed over the area externally also helps, as does eating garlic. Diet should be aimed toward efficient elimination and blood purification. Begin with a seven-day grapefruit fast or carrot juice fast.

....

Seek the advice of a qualified practitioner before fasting while you are pregnant.

....

Alternatively spend a week on raw fruit. The diet should then be entirely vegan with plenty of sprouted seeds and large portions of steamed onions. After 10 days on this blood purification regime the problem should be greatly alleviated. All sugar, refined carbohydrates, fried foods, coffee, tea, alcohol and cigarettes should be avoided.

Elevate the bed 4 in (10 cm) if the thrombosis is in the leg and avoid prolonged sitting, inactivity, crossing the legs, any form of restricted clothing and, of course, constipation. Vitamin E is an antithrombotic agent and rutin will help to strengthen the blood vessels. Evening primrose oil or borage oil will help decrease platelet adhesion, as will garlic and ginger. Lecithin, two heaped teaspoons a day, helps inhibit clotting.

PHLEBITIS FORMULA

> *Take a mixture of the following herbs:*
> *Three parts of:*
> *lime flowers*
>
> *One part of:*
> *buckwheat*
> *horse chestnut*
> *yarrow.*
>
> *Take two size 0 capsules of the finely powdered herbs with a wine glassful of decocted ginger tea with each meal.*

Note: all the above therapies are mostly for use with superficial venous phlebitis.

....

Phlebothrombosis of a deep vein is a life-threatening situation and needs immediate medical intervention.

....

STROKE

It is believed that the improved intake of vitamin C is connected to the falling incidence of stroke since the Second World War. Certainly a lack of vitamin C results in easy bruising and bleeding and this, together with high blood pressure, increases stroke risk, so ensure a good supply of fresh fruit and vegetables every day and take 1 g of vitamin C. Vitamin B complex and vitamin E may also help certain risk factors in individual patients but these need to be individually ascertained by a knowledgeable practitioner.

The natural salicylates which are richly present in apples, apricots, avocados, all berries, cherries, currants, dates, figs, grapes and raisins, grapefruit, guavas, lemons, lychees, mandarins, melons, nectarines and peaches, oranges, passion fruit, pears with their skins on, persimmons, pineapple, plums, prunes and rhubarb will reduce blood stickiness and stroke risk. The following herbs are extremely high in salicylates: aniseed, cayenne, celery seed, cinnamon, cumin, fenugreek, liquorice, mace, mustard, oregano, paprika, rosemary, sage, tarragon, thyme, white willow bark, yucca.

HEART TONIC FORMULA

> *This strengthens the heart muscle over a period of time, deplaques arterial deposits, acts as a gentle diuretic, improves blood pressure, increases peripheral circulation and strengthens the nervous system.*
> *Three parts of:*
> *hawthorn berry, leaf and flower*
> *One part of:*
> *motherwort flowers*
> *cayenne pepper*

comfrey root
garlic bulb
Siberian ginseng root
ginger root.

Make up in tincture form and give 25 to 50 drops four to five times daily, depending on the severity of the problem.

HEARTBURN SEE GASTRITIS

HEPATITIS

Also known as jaundice, this is inflammation of the liver due to infection or toxic substances. Infection can be the result of a virus, bacteria or parasites. Toxins can include antibiotics, industrial solvents and anaesthetics. The symptoms generally start with a feeling of weakness, or occasionally nausea, and often include fever and headache. The liver is tender and enlarged, the appetite poor and the sufferer is often depressed. The liver may develop cirrhosis which, in severe cases, can be fatal. As a general rule, it is only possible to get hepatitis when your resistance is low.

In both infectious and serum hepatitis faeces and blood are infectious and both types may therefore be spread by the faecal or oral route. A healthy system will generally combat such invasions, but a poor diet will often leave the liver more susceptible to infection by clogging it with unnecessary chemicals or toxins which must then be detoxified by supplying it with sufficient nutrients. Gall bladder malfunction and liver toxaemia are also major causes of degraded liver vitality.

Generally I treat hepatitis with short liver cleansing diets high in easily digestible protein such as tofu, soya beans and spirulina. The diet should also contain foods which are rich in chlorophyll, like raw and cooked green vegetables. Acute hepatitis can be combated with large doses of vitamin C, and the B complex vitamins are also important (lecithin is particularly useful as a food and food supplement).

Coffee enemas every day, alternate hot and cold compresses over the liver, plenty of rest and natural light on the skin are all very helpful. The herbs used in liver cleansing are also useful.

This is a serious condition. Seek professional medical advice urgently.

HYPOGLYCAEMIA

This is not a disease as such but a symptom of an imbalance in the blood glucose level which manifests itself as low blood sugar. Symptoms may include any of the following:

- fatigue
- irritability
- indigestion

- headaches
- obesity
- alcoholism
- PMT
- numbness
- joint pain
- nightmares
- epilepsy
- hyperactivity
- anxiety
- forgetfulness
- breathlessness
- migraine
- vertigo
- food cravings
- blurred vision
- a lack of sex drive
- fainting and blackouts
- angina
- neuralgia
- stomach cramps
- depression
- panic feelings
- sweating
- phobias
- cold extremities
- allergies
- tinnitus
- stomach ulcers.

At some time in their lives most people experience one or more of these symptoms. This is usually due to transient hypoglycaemia which may be defined as a temporary or passing drop in blood sugar level. This is soon rectified by the body's own sugar regulatory mechanism. So once a balance is achieved the symptoms usually fade. If however there is a real long-term imbalance in sugar regulation, the symptoms may well change but they will always return unless the imbalance is corrected.

There are three kinds of hypoglycaemia: severe, diabetic and reactive. Blood sugar level is normally confined within a safe narrow range of variation by the hormone insulin secreted by the pancreas which reacts quickly to even the most subtle changes. Too much insulin results in too much sugar being driven into the cells and as a consequence a steep drop in blood sugar, which particularly affects the normal function of the brain. Seek professional advice if symptoms are severe.

Causes of hypoglycaemia include too much refined carbohydrate, chronic stress, food intolerance, thyroid problems, deficiencies of vitamin B complex, chromium, manganese, zinc, potassium and magnesium, skipped meals, excessive tea and coffee drinking, cigarettes and alcohol.

TREATMENT

Take six small meals of unrefined foods which are digested slowly. Avoid dried fruits and all fruit juices as well as salt, tea, coffee and alcohol and, of course, cigarettes. Eat fresh fruit with a small amount of protein like yogurt and nuts. The only exception to this rule is bananas which are extremely high in sugar. Well-ripened ones may be eaten very occasionally once the treatment has continued for some months. Use only whole grains. Dairy products are fine if you do not have any intolerance and avocados and nutritional yeast are especially helpful. Natural honey needs to be used very moderately. A tub of yogurt with four teaspoons of nutritional yeast is a good idea just before bed, to prevent blood sugar starvation while sleeping.

Fenugreek, dandelion root and liquorice are specifics for hypoglycaemia but the prolonged use of goldenseal may actually cause hypoglycaemic symptoms. Fenugreek must be used sparingly and warily – never more than three wine glassfuls a day – and only for a short period of time, not longer than four weeks at any one stretch. In the middle of a crisis drink a decoction of equal parts of gentian root and dandelion root. It tastes foul but works quickly to stabilize blood sugar levels.

TEA FOR HYPOGLYCAEMIA

Take three to four cups daily of a decoction of the following tea, and do not let it stand around or it will turn to an unappetizing jelly because of the mucilage of the fenugreek.
Three parts of:
dandelion root
Two parts of:
comfrey root
Siberian ginseng
mullein
One part of:
fenugreek
liquorice
saffron.

After four weeks substitute one part of fenugreek with one part of kelp. Exercise initially should be gentle and sustained until a noticeable improvement is felt, at which time it should become gradually more vigorous.

Gentle walking and lots of deep breathing are the best form of exercise at the beginning of treatment.

IMPETIGO

This is a highly infectious bacterial disease which produces yellow crusting patches on the skin. Scrupulous hygiene is absolutely essential. As with all infection, impetigo usually only occurs when the person concerned is run down so take plenty of the Superfoods (see page 18) and ensure that there is an abundance of easily digestible protein in the diet. Diet and its effect on immunity and general well-being is a significant factor in staphylococcal infections such as this. Fruit juice fasting, because it is naturally so high in sugar, is contraindicated in this instance. Ensure that there are plenty of vegetables, particularly dark green leafy ones, in the diet and severely restrict the amount of fruit eaten and fruit juice drunk.

Wash the area thoroughly with diluted tincture of goldenseal and apply the diluted tincture in compresses to adherent crusts which should be removed for rapid healing. Apply tea-tree oil at full strength on the infection and repeat every two waking hours. If the skin is so raw that this is going to cause too much pain, use a poultice of three parts of castor oil to half a part of eucalyptus. Change pillow covers, sheets and towels nightly and boil anything that comes in touch with the impetigo. Take the liver flush on page 80 with at least three cloves of garlic added. Alter the dose accordingly for children depending on age (see page 61).

IMPOTENCE AND FRIGIDITY

Frigidity, nymphomania and impotence are vague terms which do not have any precise meaning. Once a woman is labelled frigid, however, or a man impotent, or worse still if such terms are self-inflicted, the person concerned naturally becomes anxious, inadequate, helpless and hopeless. No woman is frigid and no man impotent. All men, given time, patience and counselling, can maintain an erection and control ejaculation. Similarly, a woman given understanding, sympathy and gentle coaching through exploratory exercises by herself, and then with her partner, can not only enjoy sex, but can reach orgasm without too much difficulty.

The only real prerequisite is loving your partner. If you don't, or your partner does not excite you sexually, nothing on earth is going to solve your problems. No amount of sexual counselling, sexual therapy, experimentation and exercises will mend the rift between you if feeling has gone.

During the sexual excitement phase a woman's uterus, vagina, clitoris and vulva fill with blood and swell until they reach a state of vasocongestion, which often causes tension and pressure. Some doctors have insisted that this can only be relieved by orgasm but in fact exercise, cold showers and the passage of time will do the same thing, though not as pleasurably of course! There is no real clinical evidence that proves that pelvic congestion can lead to serious health problems. So let's scotch the myth that a woman must have an orgasm in order to be healthy and if she doesn't something is wrong.

But if it is orgasms you want, bear in mind that the single most common cause of a woman failing to reach orgasm is inadequate stimulation, although there are other possibilities – underdevelopment of the endocrine and nervous system, diabetes, fear or ignorance, or immaturity of the female or male genitalia.

Impotence in men has many causes but it often related to an enlarged prostate, so if this is a problem, see it as a warning of incipient prostate enlargement and get this checked. Other factors such as very bad vitamin deficiencies or heavy metal poisoning may affect sexual performance. Remember too that many prescription drugs have impotence or frigidity as a side effect; they include Aldomet, Bentyl, Hydropes, Inderal and Reserpine.

Physical and physiological causes will of course need to be looked at individually.

Alternating hot and cold sitz-baths taken twice daily are excellent, as are icy-cold plunges up to the waist after a sauna. It is advisable to detoxify the body so begin with an initial fast for three or four days on fruit or vegetable juices and follow this with a diet of fruit, vegetables, nuts, grains and seeds to further detoxify the body.

Avoid hormones in animal products. Modern animal rearing now involves administering hormones to animals in the form of ear implants. One of these hormones, zeranol, is a form of oestrogen made from fusarium. This hormone occurs naturally in crops cut in damp weather and, given our miserable climate, the level of this hormone in our food can be quite high.

A large percentage of women in Britain are noticeably zinc deficient and some animals ingest copper-containing formulae which makes this balance even worse because copper is antagonistic to zinc. A copper IUD is not advisable for this reason. A zinc deficiency can be responsible for impotence, infertility and low sperm count, and reduced sex drive. Because zinc supplementation can reduce interaction with other dietary elements, do not take at mealtimes.

Anyone taking long-term steroids, penicillin or diuretics and all alcoholics need to have their zinc status regularly monitored.

The following tonics may help.

FEMALE TONIC

Equal parts of:
chaste tree berries
wild yam
dong quai
damiana
liquorice
hops.

Take 70 drops of the tincture four times a day.

MALE TONIC

> Equal parts of:
> saw palmetto
> Korean ginseng
> Siberian ginseng
> sarsaparilla
> oats
> kola nut
> ginger.

Take 70 drops of the tincture three times a day.

This formulation is particularly helpful for men who feel they have lost their edge and their male drive. It stimulates male energy and sexual desire and will promote more frequent harder erections for longer durations as well as increasing sperm count.

INCONTINENCE

This is an enormously widespread problem among the middle aged and elderly but is one of those subjects which is simply not discussed. When I brought it into the public arena on a television programme some years ago, the switchboard was flooded with more queries about what I was saying than any other topic they ever had discussed in that station.

Incontinence can be caused by a number of physical and psychological factors, including obstetrical trauma, poor pelvic-floor tone, neglecting pre- and postnatal exercises, obesity, a swollen prostate gland and increased inter-abdominal pressure. Far too much surgery is performed to help correct incontinence and most of it could be prevented by simply carrying out prenatal and postnatal exercises faithfully.

Pelvic exercise should begin in early pregnancy (if not before) and continue after the birth regularly for at least three months or longer. Dr Arnold Kegel, professor of obstetrics and gynaecology at the University of California in Los Angeles, was the first man to popularize the necessity of pelvic-floor exercises in preventing and treating incontinence. The pelvic-floor group of muscles helps to support the pelvic contents and when contracted restrains urine flow and prevents bowel movements. Women's anal sphincter muscles are generally very strong so they need to concentrate on the vaginal and urethral sphincters to help exercise the pelvic-floor muscles.

- Practise slowing urine flow and eventually stopping it to gain a sense of which muscles are involved. As you get better at this, practise stopping urine flow, holding it for one to two seconds, and repeat six to eight times as you urinate but never do this with your first morning urination. Eventually you will find you should be able to stop urine flow quickly without any leakage and that you can slowly relax the pelvic-floor muscles in stages from full contraction to full relaxation.

- Using the same muscles, contract the pelvic floor throughout the day. Do this whenever and wherever possible but it should be repeated six to eight times during each session, building up to 100 times a day. Hold the contraction two to five seconds and then relax.
- Contract the pelvic-floor muscles while making love. Ask your partner to tell you when he can feel the difference. Repeat many times whenever the opportunity arises.

Note: While doing these exercises, remember not to hold your breath, bear down or contract the bottom, inner thighs or abdominal muscles. Far better to learn to localize the contraction to the pelvic-floor muscles entirely and do not exhaust the pelvic-floor muscles in the early stages of your learning. Do as many contractions at a time as you can do at your maximum contraction and then add two more.

Swimming using the breaststroke will help build up pelvic-floor muscles as will abdominal exercises and alternate hot and cold sitz-baths. Take the kidney bladder tonic and the kidney bladder tea on page 85. You need to do this over a period of several months for it to have good effect.

INDIGESTION SEE GASTRITIS

INFERTILITY

About 25% of all couples conceive the first month they try; 50% will have succeeded within six months, and 85% within a year. Of the remaining 15%, one quarter will conceive in the following year.

MALE INFERTILITY

In about 40% of these cases the problem is due to the male partner and usually the trouble is one of low sperm count. An increasing number of articles state that the quality of modern sperm is being heavily affected by insecticides. Other factors which impair sperm production can be heavy metal poisoning, radiation exposure (including X-rays) or prolonged drug use, both recreational and prescribed drugs, as well as an undetected infection leading to atrophy of the testicles, or a trauma or blow to the testicles. Sometimes a serious case of adult mumps will affect fertility, as will kidney failure, chronic lung disease (usually from smoking), thyroid deficiency and calcium, Vitamin E or zinc deficiency. A low sperm count has been detected in regular drinkers of alcohol. Obstruction of the seminal tract itself may be congenital or due to inflammation of the prostate, inflammation of the testicles or any other local inflammatory process, as well as more widespread infections of the kidneys or liver.

With repeated ejaculations the number of sperm in the ejaculate declines, so if your partner has ejaculated several times over the preceding few days, conception is less likely to occur on the day you ovulate because his semen will contain insufficient sperm. For this reason it is probably best to abstain from intercourse for two to three days before ovulation is expected to occur.

If a woman stands up and walks around immediately after making love, most of the seminal fluid will leak out of her vagina. To give as many sperm as possible a chance of reaching the Fallopian tubes where the egg will be, it is a good idea to lie on the bed for at least 20 minutes after making love with your bottom raised up slightly on a pillow and the knees bent in toward the chest.

One-fifth of those men who are infertile are found to produce high levels of superoxide radicals in their semen and vitamin E, which acts as an antioxidant, will mop these up. Infertile men should also realize that sperm cannot be manufactured in excessive heat. This includes heat from very hot showers, baths, saunas, Turkish baths, as well as tight-fitting underwear and trousers or electric blankets at night. Underwear should be loose – boxer shorts are ideal – and cotton, and cold showers as well as cold sitz-baths on a twice daily basis are an excellent idea, particularly before intercourse.

Smoking decreases a man's sexual capability by damaging the minute blood vessels that supply blood to the penis, so the obvious solution is to stop smoking. Studies in North Carolina in the United States show that drinking four cups of coffee a day and smoking more than 20 cigarettes was a dangerous combination for male fertility. Margarine has also been implicated in low sperm counts; sperm of an inappropriate consistency can be corrected by large doses of vitamin C. The classic herbs for correcting male infertility are gotu kola, damiana and saw palmetto. To any formulation I normally also like to add prickly ash and a touch of cayenne pepper to assist the circulation.

FEMALE INFERTILITY

A very common cause of female infertility is blocked or partly blocked Fallopian tubes which can be the result of previously undetected pelvic infections, particularly chlamydia. Some women develop antibodies to their partner's sperm, part of an allergic reaction, and this can be corrected by having your partner use a condom for three months during which time your own antibodies will decrease. Other causes of infertility include failure to ovulate, tension, stress and tiredness, cervical polyps, inflammation of the cervix or ovaries, fibroids, ovarian cysts, endometriosis and failure to orgasm during intercourse. The strong muscular contractions of a female orgasm help to push sperm from the uterus into the Fallopian tubes where eggs are fertilized; aided by these contractions sperm can travel this distance in a mere 15 minutes.

While male impotence has always been an obvious factor in infertility, until recent studies at the Hammersmith Hospital in London, female impotence – or the inability to achieve an orgasm – had not been on the agenda. When infertility in a woman is described as idiopathic, meaning no one knows the cause for certain, this aspect of infertility might well be worth considering.

The pill and STDs affect fertility as do vitamin E deficiency, diabetes and steroids. Apparently, women whose mothers smoked when they were pregnant are only 50% as fertile as women who were not exposed in this way *in utero* and when working with infertile couples I always check the possibility of heavy metal intoxication as well as B_{12} and iron deficiencies.

OVULATION TIMING SELF TEST

If you are under 30 and have been trying to conceive for more than six months without success, check that you are not consistently making love on infertile days of the month. You can do this by using a temperature chart, detecting the change in your cervical mucus, or using a chemically impregnated dipstick to detect the LH in your urine samples (for availability see Resources Directory). While your natural fertility tends to decline after the age of 30, if you have had a child or a previous pregnancy and are unable to conceive, you and your partner may be advised to have a complete diagnostic evaluation. Be warned: the diagnostic tests that specialists use may include using tubes, needles or viewing instruments, radiation, anaesthetics and dye materials.

INFERTILITY DRUGS

Some drugs used to treat infertility can cause problems. Clomid, for example, causes flushes in 10% of the women who use it and ovarian enlargement in 14%. Other side effects include blurred vision, double vision, spots in front of the eyes, after-images, sensitivity to artificial light, floaters, waves, cataracts, detachment of the posterior vitreous, spasming of the blood vessels, thrombosis of the retinal arteries, abdominal distention, pelvic pain, nausea and vomiting, increased appetite, constipation, diarrhoea, breast discomfort, abnormal menstrual bleeding, dryness of the vagina, headaches, dizziness, lightheadedness, vertigo, nervous tension, insomnia and fatigue, depression, increased urinary frequency and skin rashes, hair loss, hair dryness, weight gain or weight loss, jaundice and fluid in the abdomen.

Clomid taken by women who were already pregnant has jeopardized the health of the baby *in utero*, including the potential for congenital heart disease, Down's syndrome, club foot, congenital intestinal conditions, abnormal position of the urethra or its opening, a small head, harelip, cleft palate, congenital hip displacement, birthmarks, undescended testicles, extra fingers, conjoined twins, inguinal hernia, umbilical hernia, fused fingers, funnel chest, muscle disorders, dermoid cysts, spina bifida and other defects. There is also the potential for multiple births.

All other fertility drugs contain risks both to the baby and yourself on about the same level. Robert Mendelsohn advises staying away from fertility drugs for very good reasons. You always have the choice. My first option would always be to try the natural way before getting involved in the more problematical chemical alternatives.

HOLISTIC TREATMENT

Too many infertile couples think only of their reproductive organs, when the problem is likely to be far more wide-ranging. I have had a huge amount of success in this area by using a holistic approach. I begin with the supposition that nature cannot sprout healthy seed in unhealthy soil so treatment normally includes systematic detoxification. Which systems need detoxifying is determined by an iridology test. In both sexes an inadequate flow of energy circulating through the reproductive organs will depress fertility and this is often due to imbalances in hormones caused by poor diet and a stressful lifestyle. The treatment I use may sound radical to some but I have a very high rate of success and a wall covered in pictures of babies which doctors and specialists pronounced were impossible, a source of deep joy and satisfaction to me.

Systemic detoxification is discussed fully in my *Holistic Woman's Herbal* (Bloomsbury, 1995). Basically, it includes short vegetable juice fasts of five consecutive days every fortnight with a vegan diet in between including plenty of raw and sprouted foods. Sometimes I insist that this diet remains totally raw and organic for the first month or two and, while systemic detoxification is going on, I suggest using barrier methods of contraception to prevent the possibility of conception. Alcohol, tea, coffee, sugar and salt should be removed from the diet altogether, and I encourage the use of as much organic produce as possible, particularly pre-soaked and low-heated grains and sprouted grains and beans and seeds; all water should be filtered. I often use specific Superfoods like spirulina, chlorella, beetroot powder, purple dulse, the inner peels from oranges and lemons, rose hips, and so on, depending on the outcome of the vega or iridology test. I nearly always begin by cleaning out the bowels of both partners, and then I suggest endocrine balances including motherwort, agnus castus, false unicorn, dong quai, red raspberry, squawvine, blessed thistle, wild yam and fennel. These are particularly useful in the case of hormone imbalance. I make a good female fertility tonic which includes equal parts of damiana, wild yam, liquorice, Siberian ginseng, oat seed, gota kola, ginger, false unicorn, agnus castus and motherwort. The herbs are finely powdered and mixed together and the dose is two capsules three times a day with meals.

George Wooton, an MD practising in Hurley, New York, runs a programme that is more radical than mine and claims close to 100% success. His programme consists of a five-day fast on nothing but purified water together with rigorous bowel cleansing beginning from the third day, then three more weeks of raw fruits and vegetables only. He suggests that on this programme alone, nearly all of the people he has treated are pregnant within three to four months.

INSECT BITES AND STINGS

Remove the sting by flicking it out with the thumbnail so the barb comes out cleanly without tearing the skin and, if one is to hand, rub the area with a cube of ice. Alternatively, suck up and spit out the poisons. Rub a pulped leaf of ivy, plantain or a piece of raw onion on to the sting. Apply a salt water compress with a little tincture of ivy or plantain added to the area that has been stung. Take 10 drops of tincture of plantain every hour internally until the swelling and itching have subsided completely.

FOR A STING IN THE THROAT

To prevent choking, gargle frequently with four teaspoons of salt in a cup of water. If tincture of plantain is available add 10 drops to the water. Once the poison has been partly drawn out by the salt water gargle, apply a cabbage leaf poultice externally to the neck (see page 44).

INSECT REPELLENTS

To repel insects eat plenty of garlic or nutritional yeast.

DR CHRISTOPHER'S INSECT REPELLENT

Equal parts of:
rosemary
basil
wormwood
rue.

Crush the herbs together well in a pestle and mortar and pour over olive oil (preferably organic) in proportions of one part of herbs to five parts of oil. Add 1 dessertspoon of cider vinegar and cover the bowl. Set it over a radiator for a week. Strain well while the moisture is warm. Measure out the oil and repeat in proportions one part of fresh herbs added to five parts of the oil. Do this two more times and on the third time let the mixture sit over the radiator for at least a couple of weeks. Strain well. You will now have an extremely effective concentrated oil which will keep insects away and is good for the skin at the same time. A little of it dabbed on to the insect sting quickly helps the swelling and itching go away.

Dr Christopher's insect repellent is preferable to the citronella oil used in natural commercially marketed preparations. Citronella smells so nasty it acts as a human repellent, not just an insect one!

INSOMNIA

The first and most important prerequisite in beating insomnia is daily exercise. If you do not exercise on a regular basis, the acetyl choline will build up to such an extent that your nervous system will become fogged with it, making you irritable and jumpy. Aerobic exercise (and remember you can reach an aerobic level simply by walking briskly) is the only exercise that will burn this off. Exercise outdoors is better than inside and you will have noticed yourself how a day spent outdoors in a park or on a beach makes you feel very tired when your return home.

Skin brushing followed by alternate hot and cold showers, especially on the head, is a wonderful way to calm the nervous system (see pages 51 and 87). It should not be done just before bed as it will keep you awake. Walking barefoot on soil or grass just before going to bed helps, by releasing the excessive electrical charge built up in the body during the course of the day while walking on synthetic surfaces and literally grounding it into the natural substance beneath your feet. Aim to walk barefoot on grass, sand or soil for five minutes a day and dry your feet vigorously afterward with a rough towel, then slip them into warm socks followed by shoes or slippers. Ideally this should be done just before bed. If you don't have a garden, try going to bed in a pair of loose-fitting wet cotton socks covered by a large pair of woollen socks (unless you are prone to athlete's foot). This sounds odd and uncomfortable but actually it isn't and it does induce sleep. Ensure that you sleep in natural clothing and 100% cotton sheets. Before going to bed take a bath at 94–97°F 34–36°C with 10 drops of camomile oil added to the bath water. This will help to reduce congestion of the brain and spinal cord. Sleep with your window slightly ajar at night or have an ionizer plugged into your bedside at night.

Experiments in America have proved that paradoxical intention may be helpful for chronic insomniacs. This means doing the opposite of what you want to make it happen. For example, in one experiment insomniacs were asked to stay awake as long as possible in order to note their insomniac thoughts. One woman reduced her wakeful periods from 90 minutes to five and a half minutes! Go to bed only when you are tired and once there do not watch television. (Indeed you should not have a television set in your bedroom because of the electromagnetic fields around it.) Do not read or lie awake worrying. If you do not fall asleep quickly get up, go out of the bedroom and do something until you feel ready to try again. Eat lightly before going to bed. Set the alarm for the same time every morning, including weekends. Several cups of valerian tea sweetened with honey may be helpful or you could try one valeriana comp tablet taken at the same time each night; if necessary, increase the dose to two. They are extremely effective (see Resources Directory).

IRRITABLE BOWEL SYNDROME

Spastic colon, or irritable bowel syndrome, is three times as common among women as men. Bowel movements will alternate between bouts of constipation and diarrhoea usually accompanied by flatulence and distension. Unsurprisingly this is often accompanied by tiredness, depression, anxiety and irritability. Irritable bowel syndrome is common with post-viral fatigue but may also be the result of stress, lack of digestive enzymes, spastic bowel tone and a wide range of food intolerances, especially to dairy products, the gluten in wheat and other grains, oranges and coffee, as well as an inability to digest roughage. If the latter is the case restrict whole grains and whole grain products and use the Intestinal Corrective Formulation No. 3 on page 152; this will iron out bouts of constipation and help smooth bowel movements. Be sure to take plenty of juice with it and water following it. The abdominal exercises on the slant board (see page 168) and the Kegel pelvic exercises (see page 182), as well as yoga, will help to strengthen and tone the area and promote normal intestinal contractions. If the intake of antibiotics has upset the bacterial flora in the intestines and interfered with the proper digestion of food, take plenty of bioacidophilus (see Resources Directory). Take two tablespoons twice daily of pure aloe vera juice (see Resources Directory). Use if necessary a finely orchestrated combination of Intestinal Corrective formulations Nos. 1 and 3 together (see pages 142 and 144). Wild yam tincture taken as often as needed will help to stop spasm and calm wind.

In an acute attack try a camomile compress on the abdomen. Lie down and cover it with a large dry towel and wrap all over with a thick flannel or blanket. Colonic irrigation on a regular basis with a professional therapist for a month or two can also be very helpful.

....

Note: Irritable bowel syndrome can be caused by appendicitis so it is important that if there are any doubts as to the origin of the symptoms and pain, a doctor is consulted without delay.

....

JAUNDICE SEE HEPATITIS

JETLAG

Jetlag only arises on crossing one or more time zones, when the body resists adjusting to new cycles of sleep and wakefulness. There are no effects of jetlag on north–south flights.

Adjust as soon as you board the plane. If by your calculations it will be night when you land, pull down your window blind, wear a sleep mask and try to sleep if possible. If you need some help, take the valeriana comp mentioned for insomnia (see page 188). If you leave at night and will be arriving during the day, try to keep awake, with your eyes open and the seat light on, to make it seem as if you are already in the new time zone. Reset your watch immediately after take off because it will help you to get into tune with the new periods of day and night you will have to adjust to on arrival.

If you land in daylight, do not give in to the temptation to go to your hotel and take a nap. This will only encourage your old rhythms to keep working. Stay outdoors in natural light if possible. If you are indoors, keep the lights on and stay awake. If you arrive at night, go straight to your hotel room and try and sleep.

Diet is vital. Protein-rich foods can provide up to five hours of energy whereas foods which are high in carbohydrate such as pasta, salad, fruit and rich desserts provide an hour's energy surge but then tend to make you drowsy. If you arrive at your destination in the morning after a long flight and need to get down to work without delay, start with a high-protein breakfast and eat a high-protein lunch to keep you going through the afternoon. For dinner eat carbohydrates to ensure sleep.

Aromatherapist Daniele Ryman stocks an excellent range of aromatherapy oils for jetlag which are now being successfully used by the pilots who fly for New Zealand Airlines (see Resources Directory).

KIDNEY DISEASE

Nephritis is a serious disease of the kidneys and requires the expert attention of a qualified medical herbalist well versed in its treatment. There are many herbs which actually irritate a diseased kidney, hence the need for expert help. Chronic cases may take two to three years to heal but I have worked very successfully with this condition. The worse cases I have tried to help are those which have been treated with almost non-stop courses of antibiotics over a prolonged period of time.

KIDNEY STONES

These stones are usually made of calcium oxalate but some stones contain urates, phosphates, or cystine and it is important that the practitioner treating them knows what type of stone is present in order to ensure success. Certain stones are caused by kidney disease and there are many dietary factors that increase the risk of kidney-stone formation including refined carbohydrates, particularly sugar, which can increase the absorption of calcium from the gut and elevate its level in the urine of certain prone individuals. Vegetarians have a lower risk of forming kidney stones due to the lower incidence of uric and oxalic acid, both of which are involved in stone formation. People who consume large quantities of calcium-containing antacids together with milk as they attempt to soothe indigestion or peptic ulcers also risk developing high blood-calcium levels and so kidney stones. Alcohol, salt, and the oxalic acid naturally occurring in certain foods like tea, coffee, chocolate, peanuts, spinach, rhubarb and beetroot can also aggravate stone formation.

No matter what type of stone you have, you should eat plenty of dietary fibre. Wheat and bran both reduce calcium absorption. Eliminate animal proteins, especially meat, and cut out milk. (There are far superior sources of calcium including carrot juice, tahini – (a sesame-seed paste readily available from health-food shops), sardines, millet, oats and all dark green leafy vegetables.) Avoid refined carbohydrates, particularly those that are sugary. Drink plenty of mineral water. Reduce alcohol consumption and cut out salt altogether. Those with oxalate-containing stones or high oxalate levels in the urine should avoid food rich in oxalate acid. In such instances B_6 and magnesium may also be useful. B_6 controls the body's production of oxalic acid increasing oxalate secretion, while magnesium helps increase the solubility of oxalate in the urine. Both of these are richly present in nutritional yeast.

EMERGENCIES

Apply a poultice of hops, mullein and lobelia (available only from a qualified medical herbalist), as hot as possible, to the kidneys if pain is severe. Keep the poultice in place with a hot water bottle and leave for one hour. If after this time the pain still persists, administer an enema of goldenrod tea. You are unlikely to be able to take anything by mouth during the course of a severe attack. Sit in a hot sitz-bath for half an hour, applying a cold compress to the wrist and another cold compress to the forehead. While doing so massage the stomach lightly downward from the navel to the pubic hairline, which will help to gently move the stone into the bladder. Then get out of the bath and apply a herbal poultice for a further hour, repeating this process until such time that the stone has passed into the bladder. If you feel like drinking, take a little plantain tea.

Note: This treatment is best supervised by a consultant medical herbalist.

Follow-up treatment includes alternate hot and cold sitz-baths because the stone must not be allowed to remain in the bladder. This, together with plantain tea, will help to remove it (the only need for a surgical operation is if the size of the stone defies natural physical measures).

TEA FOR THE KIDNEYS

This is a good general maintenance tea to be drunk as a preventative.
Equal parts of:
hydrangea root
gravel root
marshmallow root.

Drink three cups decocted daily with meals. If there is any hint of infection add three parts of echinacea to this mixture and increase the dose to six cups daily.

LEG CRAMPS SEE CRAMPS
LEG ULCERS SEE VARICOSE VEINS
LIVER SPOTS

These are large brown freckles which usually appear on the back of hands and seem to be the result of age and lack of vitamins E, C and B_2. Massage nightly with cold-pressed castor oil. If this is done on a regular basis it will achieve extremely good results.

LUMBAGO SEE BACK PAIN
MASTITIS

This is the result of inflammation of the breast and milk duct system due to infection by the staphylococci. It can be the result of improper nipple preparation prior to lactation, a shallow grip on the nipple by the baby, incomplete emptying on feeding, an engorged breast, a nipple fissure which has become infected or poor nipple care and hygiene. It generally occurs during lactation but it is possible to get mastitis when not breastfeeding.

PREPARING THE BREASTS FOR BREASTFEEDING

The second trimester is the ideal time to begin to minimize the chances of sore, cracked or bleeding nipples by exposing them to the sun on a regular basis and by massaging them with the following oil. (You do not need to stand right up to the window's edge, but can be halfway into the room; the natural sunlight will stream in and help.)

BREAST AND BELLY OIL

4 oz (115 g) coconut butter
1 oz (30 ml) almond or olive oil
3 teaspoons grated beeswax (or vitamin E oil)
50 drops lavender oil (optional)
25 drops neroli oil (optional)

Melt all the ingredients together in a double boiler and begin to massage your legs, belly and breasts at least once daily with this glorious smelling mixture.

Skin brushing the breasts is also particularly helpful (see page 87) and gently rubbing the nipples with a fairly rough flannel will stimulate them into becoming more erect and so easier for the baby to latch on to. Inverted nipples can be encouraged outward by wearing a breast shield during the last few weeks of pregnancy.

To minimize stress on the breasts during nursing, alternate them. Make sure that the baby takes enough of the nipple and the areola into his or her mouth while nursing. Insert a finger into the corner of the baby's mouth to break the baby's suction on the breast at the end of each nursing session.

INFECTION

If you get a breast infection, apply hot poultices of mullein and lobelia to the breast and make sure that you are getting plenty of calcium in the form of calcium-rich tea.

CALCIUM-RICH HERBAL TEA

Two parts of:
oat straw
One part of:
alfalfa
nettles
peppermint
horse tail
Four parts of:
raspberry leaf.

Place 1 oz (30g) of herbs in cold water and bring to a simmer over a low heat. Remove from the heat source immediately and keep the pot covered for 20 minutes or longer before straining and drinking. Aim to drink three large breakfast cups a day; sweeten if desired.

Take plenty of liquids and hot baths and get lots of rest because breast infections are often the result of exhaustion. You shouldn't suffer from any breast engorgement if you nurse from the time of birth onward. A hot ointment such as tiger balm or the deep heat oil (see Resources Directory) massaged specifically into the area that hurts can be tremendously comforting and has been very effective with my own patients.

Seek the advice of a qualified medical herbalist.

MEASLES SEE CHILDHOOD DISEASES

MÉNIÈRE'S DISEASE

This is characterized by severe vertigo, progressive deafness and tinnitus (ringing in the ears) and can sometimes be accompanied by a sensation of fullness in the ears. On autopsy oedema of the membranous labyrinth has been discovered but no one yet knows why this happens. Get a proper check-up to make sure that it is Ménière's disease because cholesteatoma has the same symptoms. Cholesteatoma is the result of a tumour growing from the middle ear into the central nervous system. Also note that excessive use of aspirin can cause exactly the same symptoms.

I have had great success with this by putting patients on a seven-day vegetable juice fast every six weeks, alternated with a mainly raw-food vegan diet. Obviously this means removing tea, coffee, chocolate, salt, fried foods, alcohol and any drugs from the diet. Brisk walking to get blood up into the brain and circulating properly is helpful, as are alternate hot and cold head showers taken morning and evening. Sometimes spinal and cranial manipulation is indicated but I have often found that simply a better diet will enable the body to heal itself.

MENOPAUSE

As Germaine Greer observed, 'Though there is no public rite of passage for the woman approaching the end of her reproductive years, there is evidence that women devise their own private ways of marking the irrevocability of the change. Menopause is a time of taking stock, of spiritual as well as physical change and it would be a pity to be unconscious of it.' The Ancient Greeks used to call the menopause the climacteric, meaning 'a step in the ladder'. They saw it as simply one of the seven-year life cycles, where gradually, gently and gracefully a woman was relieved of the burden of being able to have children.

Nature has designed the menopause to be a slow downward shift in the process of oestrogen output by the ovaries with minimal side effects. In a healthy, well-nourished active woman the pituitary gland signals the adrenal glands to increase their oestrogen output and this back-up system helps to keep a small measure of oestrogen in the circulation, thereby maintaining the secondary sexual characteristics. If the adrenal glands are exhausted as the result of poor diet, constant stress, hypoglycaemia or any other nutritional deficiency, the menopause may manifest its darker side. Symptoms may include:

- haemorrhaging
- hot flushes and cold sweating
- palpitations
- vertigo
- tingling
- chills
- nervousness
- excitability
- depression
- irritability
- fatigue
- insomnia
- headaches
- muscle and bone aches
- gastro-intestinal or urinary disturbances.

The final outcome may be:

- osteoporosis
- a frequent desire to urinate
- stress incontinence
- unwanted hair
- the drying of vaginal secretions, resulting in painful sex and vaginitis
- overweight
- dry or itching skin
- reduced breast size.

This catalogue of symptoms can be avoided if you get yourself into really good shape well before it starts.

During the menopause and as you continue to age, the diet needs to be particularly good. Anything with chemicals in it should be rigorously avoided and, if you can manage it, a vegan diet is best together with abundant portions of sprouted seeds, whole grains, royal jelly, bee pollen, bananas, carrots, potatoes, apples, cherries, plums and garlic, all of which are particularly rich in natural hormones. It is essential to ensure plenty of B and E vitamins as well as zinc and essential fatty acids in the diet. Foods rich in vitamin C and bioflavonoids are also important. As oestrogen levels in the body drop, the capillary linings become thinner and leak more readily, hence hot flushes. Three to four citrus fruits with the white pith left on eaten daily will help hot flushes. Propolis, the sticky resin leaked by leaf buds and tree barks and consequently gathered by bees to cement their hives, is particularly rich in bioflavonoids. This is available in capsule form. Much of the commercially available propolis comes from areas where bees have been fed on sugar or sipped nectar from flowers contaminated with pesticides; for uncontaminated sources see Resources Directory.

SUPERFOODS FOR THE MENOPAUSE
Vitamin E

Foods rich in vitamin E stimulate the production of oestrogen and help alleviate hot sweats. Vitamin E seems to exert a normalizing effect on oestrogen levels. It has the ability to increase the hormone output in women who are deficient in it and lowers it in those who are prone to an excess. Foods rich in vitamin E include vegetable and nut oils, green leafy vegetables and wheatgerm.

Vitamin B

Foods rich in the B complex enhance the effectiveness of oestrogenic hormones and help prevent menopausal arthritis and oedema. B complex vitamins also boost the thyroid gland, important since the whole endocrine system is intimately involved in menopausal changes. A properly functioning thyroid gland is essential for normal sex hormone production because the thyroid secretes thyroxine which has a direct stimulating effect on the sex glands. An underactive thyroid gland will lead to depleted sex glands and insufficient sex hormone output.

Seaweeds

All the seaweeds will help improve the function of the thyroid gland and help to some degree to control obesity, if weight is a problem.

Calcium and Vitamin D

A malfunctioning parathyroid gland can upset calcium and vitamin D metabolism and utilization so foods rich in easily assimilable calcium are important to support parathyroid function. Vitamin D is richly present in natural sunlight.

Vitamin C and Bioflavonoids

Foods rich in vitamin C and bioflavonoids act as detoxifiers, rejuvenators and stimulants of the thyroid and sex glands. Vitamin C also encourages the body to metabolize oestrogen and the bioflavonoids help hot flushes.

Zinc

Zinc is necessary for reproductive hormone and enzyme production, for the formation of RNA and DNA, and for the proper utilization of vitamins and minerals, especially for the metabolism of vitamin A and for the synthesis of insulin and protein.

All of these are particularly concentrated in spirulina, chlorella and nutritional yeast (see page 18), whole grains, nuts and seeds and organic fruits and vegetables.

HERBAL HELP

There are many herbs rich in natural oestrogen which will help to smooth the transition from ovarian to adrenal production of oestrogen, including wild yam, lady's slipper, passion flower, black cohosh, sarsaparilla, false unicorn, elder, liquorice, fennel, Chinese angelica, sage, hops, Siberian ginseng, motherwort, marigold, false unicorn root and chaste tree.

I have had particular success helping women through any uncomfortable menopausal symptoms with the following formulation.

HORMONE REPLACEMENT THERAPY TONIC

> *Equal parts of the tinctures of:*
> *wild yam*
> *chaste tree*
> *fennel*
> *Chinese angelica.*

The dosage is normally 40 drops morning and evening and after three months this can be reduced to 20 or 30 drops morning and evening.
This really helps maintain hormonal balance.

MENSTRUAL DISORDERS

The rhythm of a woman's menstrual cycle is finally balanced and the slightest thing can throw it out of kilter; stress is a common culprit, as are emotional disturbances such as anxiety and depression. But pregnancy is the commonest cause of missed periods so, when in doubt, have a pregnancy test. The time to actively seek professional help is when you detect a permanent change in your menstrual pattern. If you start to bleed unpredictably, especially heavily or painfully, or if your periods dry up altogether and you are not in the menopause, seek guidance.

Normally you will lose only about four tablespoons of actual blood (3 fl oz or 75 ml) over four or five days. The remaining three to four fluid ounces (75 to 100 ml) is made up of water, mucus and other fluids married with fragments of decomposing tissue from the interior of the uterus and several million epithelia cells that flake off the lining of the vagina.

ANAEMIA AND MENSTRUATION

You will need a little extra iron during menstruation, as you lose 15 to 30 mg, and nine out of ten women who have periods are actually deficient in iron. My favourite iron-rich herbs are raspberry leaves (drink a cup infused three times a day) and yellow dock, which I normally administer as a tincture, 40 drops in the morning and evenings. Because tannin will inhibit its absorption, tea and coffee should be cut out of the diet while taking this; it is more effective in a little water on an empty stomach. Foods high in iron include anything red, purple or dark green, especially beetroot. One of my favourite mixtures is two-thirds freshly pressed carrot juice, one-third beetroot, with a generous plug – about the size of half a thumb – of raw ginger juiced.

CALCIUM AND MENSTRUATION

The need for calcium increases seven-fold in the week before a period begins and the most easily ingested source of calcium is carrot juice. Drink a glass morning and evening during the course of this week. Other sources of calcium include sprouted wheat, oats, walnuts, hazelnuts, almonds, cabbage, spinach, potatoes, onions and turnips.

Magnesium acts synergistically with calcium and is richly present in many of the same foods as well as beets, dates and sweetcorn.

Only 20% of menstrual pain can be accounted for by endometriosis, a retroverted uterus or some kind of infection. In the remaining 80% it is possible that a uterine contraction feels painful because of pelvic congestion, constipation, spinal lesions which have a specific action on the pelvic organs, weak abdominal tone leading to dropped abdominal and pelvic contents and resulting in congestion, poor circulation or stress. It is not uncommon, for example, for periods to cease altogether following a severe psychological or physical trauma such as rape. Women who are fearful of getting pregnant may also create all sorts of menstrual disorders.

In this instance, we don't have to know the cause in order to alleviate the problem. In some women a hot bath and a little alcohol, or simply curling up with a hot water bottle, helps. In others ice packs applied to the abdomen and hot packs supplied to the legs and feet draw blood away from the congested area. I generally assume that the gynaecological organs in women with menstrual problems are not in good condition and immediately put women on the Female Corrective Formulation on page 214, which is specifically designed to relieve painful menstruation, cramping and irregularities by rebuilding the malfunctioning reproductive system. I also offer simple herbal teas including camomile, catnip, peppermint, cramp bark or red raspberry. These can be taken in any quantity and are more effective sipped as hot as possible. Also get an osteopath to check your spine.

Alternate hot and cold sitz-baths are an unbeatable way of removing pelvic congestion and restoring ovarian, Fallopian and uterine health. These should be taken morning and evening.

Pain immediately before menstruation suggests that the position of the womb is abnormal. This can sometimes be seen in women who are very thin where the internal fat and ligament upon which the uterus is suspended has lost its tone. A uterus which is tipped toward the spine is called 'retroverted'; one which tips toward the pelvic bone is called 'antiverted'; if it bends over itself it is called 'retroflexed'. There seems to be some sort of gynaecological obsession with uterine positioning but rest assured, a tipped uterus is not a condition to worry about. Most women's uteri point in different directions at differing periods of their lives but there are very few women who have a uterus tipped to such an extreme degree that it causes pain or makes any difference in their ability to become pregnant.

However, if the uterus is truly out of position, slant-board exercises will help (see page 168), as will the simple acts of walking, swimming or yoga. The Kegel exercises on page 182 are also invaluable.

THE COLOUR OF BLOOD

Menstrual blood that is bright red is indicative of poor assimilation of sugar and carbohydrates. If it is dark red, stringy or excessively smelly it shows that the body is overburdened with protein and you should cut back on meats, eggs and dairy products. The ideal colour of healthy menstrual blood is reddish brown and it should flow easily and freely.

EXERCISES FOR MENSTRUAL PAIN (DYSMENORRHOEA)

It is very tempting to creep into bed hugging a hot water bottle feeling sorry for yourself, but try and do at least one of the following exercises, if not the whole series.

- Lie on your back at right angles to the wall, with your buttocks as near to the wall as possible. Prop your feet up against the wall, making sure that the soles are flat and the knees a little bent. Maintain this position for five minutes.
- Move away from the wall and bring one leg up as close to your chin as you can get it, leaving the other flat on the floor. Hold the lifted leg up with your arms to take the strain and maintain that position for two minutes, then swap around using the other leg.
- Get up so that you are resting on your knees and elbows and stretching your head and arms out so that your elbows are on the ground in front of you with your head between your arms. Hold this position for two minutes. This is particularly helpful for those who have pain immediately after intercourse just before a period is due.
- The cobra. This is a yogic position in which you begin by lying face down flat on the floor and then gradually raise your head and chest without using your arms. Then, using the arms, continue to raise your trunk until your back is arched and head is bent back as far as possible with your eyes cast back looking above you. Inhale as you raise your body up and exhale when you lower your trunk to the floor. Do this slowly. Relax and repeat.
- The bow. This is a yogic posture in which you lie face down, bend your knees, grab your ankles with your hands and then release and relax. Inhale as you begin and exhale after release. If you are flexible you can also rock back and forth on your stomach in the bow position while holding your breath.
- Acupressure points will also help to relieve lower back pain. Lie face down on a hard surface and have a companion press with the flat, not the tip, of the thumb along the sides of each vertebra from the tail of the spine up to the waist. Hold each pressure point to the count of 10 and then slowly release.
- One of the most pleasant methods of relieving cramps is to have an orgasm, but masturbating in order to achieve this while you are in great pain may, understandably, be out of the question.

Sometimes severe candidiasis can cause painful or irregular periods so it is worth getting this checked out.

EXCESSIVELY HEAVY PERIODS

The shadow that looms over menorrhagia, or excessively heavy periods, is cancer, although this rarely turns out to be the case if periods are regular. Still, it is worth going for a thorough check-up to see. Bleeding between periods is much more worrying, as is bleeding straight after sexual intercourse. In these instances seek immediate medical advice. Heavy bleeding may also be a symptom of fibroids, endometriosis or pelvic infection. There may also be emotional causes for heavy bleeding, notably depression. Women who have been sterilized sometimes complain of menorrhagia.

It is worth getting your spine checked by an osteopath or a chiropractor. Reflexology can often be very successful. Sit comfortably on a couch and put your foot in your lap so that you can get at the sides. The reflexology pressure points for the genitals and female organs are around the ankle. Press on the inside of your foot with the flat of your thumb on a spot about halfway between your ankle bone and the bottom of your heel: this is the uterine point. Press on a similar spot on the outside of your foot for the ovaries. Squeezing and pinching either side of your Achilles tendon about 3 in (7.5 cm) up from your heel which will also affect the uterus. If it feels tender or hurts, go gently but don't stop. Work on these points throughout the month but not during the actual flow as this will make it even heavier.

Fasting on the first day of a heavy flow or the day before certainly helps. Take 10 drops hourly of Tormentavena (see Resources Directory). Alternatively, take between 20 to 50 drops twice a day of horsetail tincture or Bioforce's Tormenta-vena throughout the entire month and, if necessary, for several months until the bleeding is lighter. Do the liver flush on page 80. The liver plays a great part in hormonal regulation. Make sure that you have an abundance of iron and calcium in your diet.

LACK OF PERIODS

While it is common for the initial periods following the menarche to be irregular, the absence of periods (amenorrhoea) is usually the result of stress, an extreme diet (including fruitarianism) or too much exercise.

Between 40 and 60 drops of chaste tree tincture morning and evening on an empty stomach can be helpful, as can the same dosage of Chinese angelica. Other herbs which may help include blue cohosh, black cohosh, false unicorn, liquorice or holy thistle. All of these may be taken as teas.

MIGRAINE

This is more serious than a headache because it involves recurrent headaches with visual and/or gastro-intestinal disturbances so there may be nausea, vomiting and an inability to look at light. Attacks can be preceded by flashes of light, the result of intercerebral vasoconstriction, followed by severe head pain confined to one side of the head or eye due to dilation of extracerebral cranial arteries. It is important to get a correct diagnosis before proceeding with treatment since a migraine is deep seated and will take longer to heal than a headache.

I have found iridology particularly useful for ascertaining whether there is any liver congestion, intestinal toxaemia or hypoglycaemia, all of which can be the underlying cause of migraine. If I catch a migraine early enough, I use lobelia in emetic doses because the induction of vomiting often helps to abort a severe migraine. However, this herb is only available on prescription from medical herbalists. Many studies have shown that certain foods, including caffeine, sugar, yeast extracts, liver, sausages, broad beans, cheese, pickled herrings, sauerkraut, oranges, bananas, wheat, milk, chocolate and food additives, exacerbate migraines. Smoking, alcohol and the contraceptive pill also play a part in migraines.

Cranial osteopathy and osteopathy may be indicated if muscular spasm or arthritis is present. If liver congestion is indicated – I find very often it is – a three-day fast, coupled with liver detoxification, castor oil packs and liver-cleansing herbs is indicated. Intestinal toxaemia calls for fasting and enemas, and in this instance I find chicory root enemas particularly helpful. They can also be used in the early stages of a migraine and sometimes may stop it in its tracks. Other herbs which help include violet, peppermint, lavender, feverfew, rosemary, valerian root, vervain, dandelion, motherwort, centaury, ginger root and skullcap. Ginger root is taken as an antiplatelet aggregatory, and it seems the blood platelets of migraine sufferers spontaneously come together more than normal between attacks. So ginger tea taken on a regular basis may prove very helpful in these instances.

If you have the kind of migraine which is relieved by a hot water bottle placed on the face or the neck, use herbs which will assist to expand the blood vessels in the head like peppermint, lavender, rosemary or feverfew. However if you have the kind of migraine that is relieved by ice packs use valerian, skullcap or motherwort. Infuse or decoct as appropriate any of these as teas and drink three cups per day. Bioforce's Migraine complex is extremely helpful. The usual dose is 30 drops three times daily (see Resources Directory).

MISCARRIAGE

It is thought that up to 40% of all pregnancies miscarry in the very early stages and are mistaken for heavy or late menstrual cycles. Excessive bleeding, cramping and clotting which are often associated with irregular or heavy menstrual cycles are sometimes simply spontaneous miscarriages. If this happens within the very early weeks of pregnancy, low progesterone levels may be the cause. If this is the case I normally put a woman on 1,600 mg of Siberian ginseng powdered in capsules daily right through her pregnancy. Those who start to cramp later in their pregnancy over the course of the sixth or seventh month or even the eight month can take double this dose for a week or two to prevent premature birth. Your doctor can give you a test to determine whether a low progesterone level is in fact the cause of your miscarriage.

....

Note: Synthetic progesterone is not recommended as it may cause birth defects.

....

An alternative progesterone-stimulating herb is wild yam root, but in my experience it is not as effective as Siberian ginseng.

Miscarriage can also be the result of stress, an inadequate diet, trauma, weak uterine muscles or a body that is too toxic to carry a baby full term. It is for this reason I place heavy emphasis on cleansing and detoxifying to enable infertile couples to conceive and women predisposed to miscarriage to carry to full term. In many cases herbs can provide that extra nourishment and strength needed to correct the problem. Rest may help to prevent a miscarriage that is only threatening but if it is going to happen in any case, rest may make no difference to the outcome.

DR CHRISTOPHER'S ANTI-MISCARRIAGE FORMULA

I have used this formulation many many times to stop women miscarrying with a great deal of success. He designed it to do this and, if necessary, to help pass a dead foetus. It works in both cases because of the lobelia it contains: where a foetus is strong lobelia assists in healing a tearing and bleeding condition and stopping the bleeding, but if the foetus is dead and should be aborted the lobelia directs the abortion.

The formulation is:
Three parts of:
false unicorn
One part of:
lobelia (only available to qualified medical herbalists)

Use a teaspoon of this combination to a cup of boiling water, making an infusion and sipping half a cup of the strained tea every half hour. Once the bleeding has stopped, take it every hour for the rest of the day and then three times a day for the next three days.

This should not be used except under the supervision of a qualified medical herbalist.

MONONUCLEOSIS

Sometimes known as the kissing disease, but more usually known as glandular fever, mononucleosis is the result of a viral infection, generally of the lymphatic glands in the throat. It should be treated rigorously with fasting on juices (warmed if swallowing is very painful), together with 360 drops (approximately 1 tablespoon) echinacea in juice. Sip slowly over the course of the day. Repeat daily for ten days. Rest for five and then resume the cycles if necessary. A warmed poultice of equal parts of mullein and lobelia tincture generously spread on to a handkerchief in tincture form should be applied to the throat at night. This should be covered with a silk scarf. During the day equal parts of the tincture should be rubbed into the swollen glands. Once the glands have returned to normal it is advisable to follow up with a course of herbal antibiotics (two every two hours for a week), and to break the fast gradually with lots of soupy grains.

MORNING SICKNESS

If a woman comes from a family that suffers from morning sickness it will be worth her while building up her adrenal glands before she gets pregnant as adrenal exhaustion can exacerbate this condition.

ADRENAL TONIC

The following formulation will help to restore hormonal function and support the adrenal glands while regulating blood sugar and increasing the body's resistance to disease, thereby counteracting stress:

Two parts of:
Siberian ginseng
One part each of:
echinacea
wild oats
bladderwrack
gotu kola.

Take 25 drops three times a day with meals in tincture form. Stay on this formulation for at least three months before conception.

It seems that a plethora of factors contributes to morning sickness, including hypoglycaemia, low levels of B complex vitamins, fluctuating dietary needs and, particularly, a steep increase in the hormone human chorionic gonadotrophin. I found that the most useful herb here is wild yam root because it both tones and feeds the liver, and balances hormone production.

WILD YAM FORMULATION

One of my most successful formulations consists of:
Two parts of:
wild yam root
One part of:
chaste berry
One part of:
ginger root.

Decoct it in a quarter of a cup of warm tea every two hours. You may need to keep this up for several days and because it is fairly strong tasting you may want to sweeten it with a little maple syrup. Its effect may not be apparent for some time, so be patient.

It is also believed that an insufficiency of vitamin B_6 can exacerbate morning sickness, so I recommend the potassium broth with added nutritional yeast (see page 31); this is not only easy to swallow but very comforting.

My pregnant patients have found that they can balance their low blood sugar levels by keeping snacks of dry biscuits spread with a little nut butter on their bedside tables. Others have preferred popcorn. Some of my patients have had difficulty producing hydrochloric acid during the first few weeks of pregnancy and in these cases I have found digestive enzymes from pineapple and pawpaw helpful, particularly if taken when eating meals high in protein. In this instance the rules of food combining need to be meticulously applied.

In rare cases where nothing seems to stay down, I have found miso soup mixed with slippery elm into a thin gruel helpful, as well as soothing and quite palatable. Miso soup can be bought ready made from health-food stores or it can be reconstituted from its dried powder form sold in packets.

One of the simplest, most delicious teas for morning sickness is ginger root tea, although it doesn't work on some people as well as the wild yam combination.

GINGER ROOT TEA

Grate 1 oz (30 g) of fresh ginger root and cover it with 1 pt (575 ml) of water. Simmer at a very low heat for 10 minutes, then strain. Add honey and lemon to taste.

This is delicious served either warm or, in hot weather, ice cold. Ginger root tea also makes a very useful formula for travel sickness, both in children and adults.

MOUTH ULCER

Rub the sore with the following lotion: six drops of essential oil of coltsfoot, three drops of tincture of myrrh, three drops of propolis. Recurrent mouth ulcers can be caused by iron, folic acid and vitamin B_{12} deficiency, all of which are richly present in nutritional yeast. Gargling nightly with warm sage tea, slushing it well around the mouth before spitting it out, will disinfect the mouth.

MULTIPLE SCLEROSIS

Mercury poisoning can produce the same symptoms as multiple sclerosis so before I begin working with a patient, I insist that they check that they haven't been poisoned by their dental amalgams (see page 95). Once this has been ruled out, I find that early symptoms of the disease can often be radically improved with changes in diet. The longer a person has had the disease the less likely a cure because the protective sheath around certain nerves becomes scarred and calcified, causing permanent damage. With prolonged and persistent treatment I have helped patients achieve very long remissions but self-discipline is of the essence.

A diet that reaps the best results is a gluten-free and dairy-free vegan diet without any saturated fats whatsoever. No tea, coffee, alcohol, salt, sugar or fried foods. I advise patients not to use gluten-free substitutes for bread-baking, but brown rice and millet are fine and I steer them away from additives and preservatives. Obviously smoking has to stop. This leaves fruits, vegetables, brown rice and millet, seeds, fermented foods such as sauerkraut washed of its salt content, cold-pressed saturated oils, nuts and nut butters, sprouted and raw seeds and all soya products.

Vitamin and mineral supplementation is often necessary and this needs to be individually tailored. Essential fatty acids and the B complex, particularly vitamin B_{13}, are specifically indicated very often. The mistake most people make is not taking enough. Evening primrose oil needs to be administered at a minimum dose of between 4.5 g and 6 g daily.

Glandular disturbances of the liver, pancreas, thyroid, adrenals and gall bladder are often part of the overall problem of multiple sclerosis and can be individually determined with an iridology test and corrected with the appro-priate herbs. Cold baths taken in warm surroundings on rising are especially helpful, preceded by vigorous skin brushing. Osteopathy with particular attention to the third and fourth cervical vertebrae and dorsals 5 and 12 is nearly always advised. Daily yoga is an excellent idea as is outdoor swimming, especially in the sea. A few of my patients have shown great improvement with hyperbaric oxygen therapy. This involves sitting in the kind of oxygen tent they put deep sea divers in for several hours at a time on a regular basis. The formulation Metasporin available from Bioforce is a good general back-up (see Resources Directory).

MUMPS SEE CHILDHOOD DISEASES

NAPPY RASH

The obvious first step in avoiding nappy rash is to allow fresh air to a baby's bottom as often as possible. Keeping your baby clean and waterproof after each bowel movement is essential. The best mixture for this is 90% jojoba oil mixed with 10% tea-tree oil. Jojoba is actually more of a wax than an oil and is extremely waterproof but easily absorbed, while tea-tree oil is anti-fungal, anti-viral and anti-bacterial.

If the rash is the result of a yeast infection you need to cut out all forms of sugar from your diet if you are breastfeeding and from your baby's diet if he or she is eating anything. Use garlic oil over the rash and make sure your baby or toddler is given appropriate probiotics. Avoid petrol-based products such as mineral oil on the baby's skin.

NEPHRITIS SEE KIDNEY DISEASE

NERVOUS BREAKDOWN SEE ANXIETY; DEPRESSION

NEURALGIA

This painful inflammation of the nerve sheaths can occur anywhere in the body where there is direct or indirect pressure on the nerves, but most usually affects the trigemminal nerve of the face. Spinal cranial manipulation may be indicated or massage or posture re-education may be helpful and your medical herbalist or naturopath will be able to determine this. Deficiencies of vitamin B_{12} can lead to neuritis and a diet which balances the acid–alkaline ratios in the body is required.

Heat applied externally is very soothing. Rub the deep heat oil directly into the skin but be sure not to get it near the eyes. Alternatively use tiger balm.

FORMULATION FOR NEURALGIA

> *The following formulation, taken internally, is useful:*
> *Equal parts of:*
> *black cohosh*
> *devil's claw*
> *cayenne*
> *ginger root*
> *wild yam.*
>
> *Take four size 0 capsules three times a day with food.*

NOSEBLEEDS

Hold the nose between the thumb and index finger and squeeze just enough to stop the bleeding but not enough to cause pain. Breath slowly while you do this through an open mouth. Hold the pressure for a minimum of five minutes without stopping. Then insert a ball of well-masticated yarrow leaf as high into each nostril as possible but not so high up that it can't be retrieved! Continue to breathe through the mouth until your nose feels comfortable and then gently extract the yarrow leaf. Alternatively, take 10 drops of cayenne tincture in a little water internally every 15 minutes until the nosebleed stops.

OBESITY

Obesity has become an epidemic in the Western world. It is the result of a particular type of malnutrition, starvation induced by ingesting empty calories, that is food with no nutritional value at all. In January 1983 the Royal College of Physicians in London confirmed that, in common with people in the USA and other Western countries, the British – particularly the young – are getting fatter, even though they are actually eating less than people did 50 years ago. Some 60% of all American children are obese and 90% cannot pass a rudimentary physical fitness test such as doing one push up. By the time Californian girls are nine, 80% of them have already been on their first diet! The burning question is not so much the quantity but quality of the food we eat.

Statistically children who are overweight by the age of two turn into fat adults more frequently than their lean playmates, so early feeding patterns set the stage for adult obesity. Most infants receive starchy food as their first solids around four months of age. This is too early for proper digestion, may set the stage for later allergies and causes rapid weight gain. Cow's milk may cause rapid weight gain because it is designed for the rapid growth of calves, rather than children. Although modulated for babies most cow's milk is homogenized, which makes the fat particles easier to assimilate. Overall breastfed infants have far less chance of becoming obese than formula-fed babies. It is, of course, essential that a breastfeeding mother is herself on an excellent diet.

Occasionally children stay thin throughout childhood because, in spite of a junk-food diet, they are getting a lot of exercise through their play; they may, however, have a history of frequent infections and possible behavioural problems. If a child becomes obese as a teenager, it may be the result not only of including alcohol in the diet, but stressing the pancreas with refined carbohydrates and sugars. This increased sugar sensitivity may then progress into a clinical case of hypoglycaemia exacerbated by the added burden of alcohol. Marry these dietary influences with the addition of stress from a job or a new family life which further depletes the adrenal glands, the co-manager of our blood sugar level along with the pancreas, and you begin to see how profoundly a body's internal chemistry can be abused.

Most obese people show abnormal glucose tolerance and have raised blood levels of cholesterol, triglycerides and free fatty acids. The fact that many obese people say that they do not eat any more than other people is often true. A thin person may simply have a different, rather than a better, biochemistry. No real progress will be made unless the actual biochemistry of an obese person is changed. For this reason I suggest that initially anyone trying to lose weight should eat only whole grains which are very lightly cooked and still chewy but not soft.

The diet should then cut out all sugars and saturated fats including natural sugar from juices. Only whole fruit should be taken. This regime should be coupled with sufficiently prolonged aerobic exercise to alter the biochemistry. Begin with 12 minutes building up to 20 to 45 five times a week minimum. Aerobic exercise includes fast walking, jogging, running, skipping, cycling, rowing, cross-country skiing, roller skating and aerobic exercise classes.

While swimming is an aerobic exercise it is not recommended for weight loss since the water temperature is usually colder than body temperature and will then signal the body to store fat for insulation, clearly not what is desired. However as a cardiovascular exercise for the entire body it is excellent. True aerobic exercise changes the body on a biochemical level, altering the deeply entrenched way anyone overweight handles carbohydrates and fats. Such exercise also stimulates the endocrine system.

A basic diet should include plenty of raw fruit but no fruit juices and limit bananas to one a day only, if desired. Plenty of raw vegetables are particularly effective if eaten at the beginning of a meal; eat fewer lightly cooked than raw. All potatoes should be eaten with the skins on, baked or steamed, but should be limited to three servings a week. Beans, sprouted seeds and sprouted beans may be taken as desired, but nuts must be restricted. You would be better off coming off animal proteins altogether while dieting. All refined carbohydrates should be avoided. Eat only conservatively cooked unrefined brown rice, barley, millet, rye, buckwheat, wheat, bulgur, corn and any other whole grains. Let your teeth do the grinding and take nothing that has been previously ground into flour for bread or cooked cereal. Use cold-pressed unsaturated oils, particularly walnut, olive and flax seed oil in moderate amounts, with lemon juice or cider vinegar for salad dressing and, when needed in cooking, in conservative amounts.

It is also far better to eat four or five smaller meals a day than two or three large ones and the main meal should be taken at midday. Eat in situations where there are no mental distractions such as television, radio or reading. You should aim to drink at least eight large glasses of water a day which will help to dilute the many toxins provided by the breakdown of proteins and fats for energy, as well as the toxins stored within the fat cells themselves which are liberated as the fat stores melt away.

Alternate hot and cold showers will stimulate the circulation in the endocrine system (see page 51). Saunas or Turkish baths should be taken several times a week. Spinal manipulation and massage may be indicated once or twice a week. The Superfoods on page 18, particularly purple dulse, spirulina and chlorella, are extremely helpful for weight loss. One of my patients lost 90 kg (200lb), by taking Fruit Smoothies with two heaped tablespoons of the Superfood stirred into it twice a day and using salads and whole grains for her third meal. Throughout, she maintained excellent health and suffered no fatigue or infections at all.

OEDEMA SEE WATER RETENTION

OSTEOPOROSIS

This abnormal porosity of the bones is usually the result of the body's inability to absorb and utilize nutrients properly, coupled with excessive consumption of protein, post-menopausal hormonal imbalances and diminished physical activity. Prolonged cortisone treatment blocks the bone-building activity and decreases the intestinal absorption of calcium, as do antibiotics. Those with rheumatoid arthritis which is being treated with steroids often have osteoporosis. Spontaneous fractures among osteoporosis sufferers are common.

The need for calcium increases in old age as the production of hydrochloric acid in the stomach dwindles, food is less thoroughly chewed because of poor teeth or dentures, and exercise tends to tail off. The richest sources of calcium are carrot juice, kelp and dark green leafy vegetables, sesame seeds and tahini, and sesame seed paste. The magnesium/calcium–phosphorus ratio in all of these items is much more balanced than those in dairy, meat or fish products and all of the minerals are more evenly metabolized. Unfortunately calcium deficiency will only manifest in X-rays after 30% of the bone is lost so it is important that women start ingesting easily absorbable sources of calcium in high quantities well before the menopause. They should not simply wait for the damage to be done. There is an excellent service in London which is available for screening of the bone mass coupled with professional advice on specifically tailored nutrition should it be indicated (see Resources Directory).

DIET

Concentrate on dark green leafy vegetables, carrots, fruits and berries of all kinds, sesame and sunflower seeds, as well as an abundance of foods rich in lactic acid, such as sauerkraut and yogurt. The best grains are oats, barley, buckwheat, millet and rice. Betaine hydrochloride tablets should be taken with each meal to assure proper assimilation, or alternatively take cider vinegar and honey in a little water before meals. Because most calcium is leached from the bones at night while the body is at rest, it is advisable to take plenty of calcium-rich foods just before bed. Any acid medium such as cider vinegar and honey will increase calcium absorption. Cut back on dairy products in order to establish proper mineral balance and cut out meat altogether because it contains 20 to 50 times more phosphorus than calcium; this aggravates calcium lost from the bones in order to keep a proper phosphorus–calcium ratio in the blood.

EXERCISE

This is vital as diminished physical activity and loss of muscle strength are contributing factors in osteoporosis. Skipping is especially recommended for its piezo-electric effect, that is its effect of generating electricity in the body. Do this in soft shoes which have a good ankle support.

HERBS

One of my patients was run over by a refuse collecting truck, which crushed most of her ribs and badly ruptured her spleen. She was already eating what in essence was a lacto-vegetarian unrefined diet, so I rushed the following formulation over to her hospital: equal parts of comfrey and horsetail, and half a part of lobelia. I asked her to take one capsule every hour with sips of nettle tea or cider vinegar and honey. Her healing was remarkable and stunned the doctors who were treating her. This is an excellent formula for mending broken bones and strengthening the thinning ones.

I would also advise a little sunbathing daily if the weather permits. Women should take the natural HRT formulation on page 196 which is rich in phyto-steroids. Unlike its synthetic counterpart, this is perfectly safe and has no side effects.

PARKINSON'S DISEASE

Like so many other difficult-to-understand degenerative diseases I have found a drastic lifestyle change and vigorous internal detoxification procedures often show remarkable results with Parkinson's disease. Such an approach certainly improves overall health. I begin by putting my patient on a month's raw food diet followed by a 14-day vegetable juice fast emphasizing carrot, beet and green vegetable juice combinations coupled with plenty of Superfoods stirred in (see page 18), and lots of potassium broth (see page 31). This fast is then broken for two days on fresh fruits. Then I put the patient back on to a raw food diet with some pre-soaked low heated grains added and plenty of nut milks. Over a period of 12 months I alternate this rejuvenation diet with periods of fasting from three to seven days every four weeks.

Sometimes heavy metal detoxification is necessary as is a careful investigation of any possible food intolerances. Forceful alternate hot and cold showers over the head help, as do foot saunas followed by cold plunges and deep muscle massage. Salt water bathing and gentle sunbathing as well as outdoor exercise are all helpful and I nearly always give lecithin as an additional supplement. The herbs I use include ginseng, damiana, prickly ash, ginger, lobelia, cramp bark, alfalfa, bayberry and Irish moss, according to individual need.

On occasion Api-cerebrum supplied by Bioforce has proved useful (see Resources Directory).

PEPTIC ULCER SEE DUODENAL ULCER

PNEUMONIA

Much depends on whether the pneumonia is bacterial, viral or bronchopneumonial; certainly bacterial pneumonia, which often starts very quickly and is very severe, needs urgent treatment with antibiotics. Viral pneumonia is generally less serious and can be treated with expert herbal management as for a fever incorporating such expectorants as thyme and lobelia.

This is not a disease to be treated by amateurs. Seek the guidance of a qualified medical herbalist urgently.

A well-managed convalescence is often essential to avoid secondary complications. During convalescence ensure deep and restful sleep in a well-ventilated bedroom and make sure the patient drinks plenty of black grape juice which oxidizes in the system without any waste and does not leach calcium from the body. Mental and emotional healing are as important as physical healing, and here the Bach Flower Remedies are of great help (see Resources Directory).

POISONING

If the victim has swallowed a poisonous food (like a toadstool) induce vomiting as quickly as possible by giving 1.5 fl oz (35 ml) of ipecacuanha syrup to an adult or 0.3 fl oz (10 ml) to a child (1 level teaspoon is 5 ml).

Do not use tincture of lobelia.

Lobelia will only speed up the digestion of any of the substance left internally. Also do not use salt water, which may induce acute salt intoxication, producing such symptoms as irritability, appetite loss, coma and convulsions. Poison centres have reported fatalities after well-meaning helpers have administered salt water.

- Vomiting can be made easier and more comfortable by taking an emetic while standing, lowering the head and rubbing the waist and abdomen gently.
- In the case of a child place the child over your knee in a spanking position with the head lower than the hips to help avoid inhalation of vomit.

Seek immediate medical help.

- If the victim has swallowed a poisonous substance several hours before and is showing symptoms of poisoning, do not waste time by inducing vomiting. Get to the hospital quickly.
- If you do not know what the victim has swallowed and he or she cannot tell you or is unconscious, ring the hospital immediately on the emergency number. Describe if possible the container and give all the information you can. They will advise you what can be done while you wait for an ambulance.
- If the substance is caustic, do not induce vomiting as it will only burn the oesophagus further. Plenty of milk will slow its absorption.
- If the patient is getting drowsy, give a double-strength decoction of peppermint tea and keep him or her walking. If the patient is unconscious do not give anything at all. Aspirin and paracetamol do not initially induce coma but in large quantities they can damage the liver so act quickly and get the patient to the hospital.

TREATMENT FOR FOOD POISONING

Administer an enema if the patient does not already have copious diarrhoea and if the food was eaten more than four hours previously. If vomiting is induced, soothe the aching stomach afterward with sips of very hot peppermint tea. The only other thing to be taken is copious amounts of mineral water served at room temperature with a squeeze of lemon juice in each glass, the more the better to combat dehydration.

Do not work against the body's natural defence process of unburdening itself by trying to stop diarrhoea, with kaolin and morphine for example. Once the patient is calmer and has stopped vomiting, give equal parts of goldenseal and chaparral two size 0 capsules every four hours. Gradually introduce pure fruit juices.

Begin as soon as possible with Bioforce's Bioacidophilus (see Resources Directory), one or two capsules every hour. This will repopulate the distressed colon with benign flora very quickly.

PREMENSTRUAL STRESS

The highest number of violent crimes committed by women take place four to seven days prior to menstruation. These days are also the peak ones for women being admitted both to prison and to psychiatric institutions and shoplifting is 30 times more common at this time. There is also a bigger percentage of female accidents and suicide attempts. In the premenstrual period brain waves are increased in frequency and amplitude compared to those of mid-cycle. These facts are proof, if proof were needed, of the true physiological and psychological alteration that takes place before a period.

Many of the physical changes of PMS are the results of a shift in fluid balance in response to progesterone which is produced in large quantities after ovulation. Physical changes may include:

- swelling of the breasts, feet and hands
- haemorrhoids
- abdominal bloating
- weight gain
- migraines
- backache
- cramping
- painful joints
- marred skin and lank hair
- asthma
- hay fever
- hoarseness
- nausea
- red eyes.

Emotional problems may include:

- food or alcohol cravings
- depression
- loss of concentration

- fatigue
- irritability.

The craving for refined carbohydrates including sugar rockets by two and a half times with PMS. It seems it is not the hypoglycaemic state itself that causes PMS because its symptoms disappear soon after food is eaten and in any case never lasts for days on end. What hypoglycaemia does is to overburden the adrenal glands as they struggle to stabilize drastically fluctuating blood sugar levels. Distressed adrenal glands need an abundance of vitamin B complex and vitamin C. These are essential for carbohydrate metabolism and are often missing in a typical Western highly refined carbohydrate diet which produces hypoglycaemia in the first place. So women with refined carbohydrate cravings get stuck in a vicious cycle, producing hypoglycaemia and adrenal exhaustion. This is why B complex and B_6 have been so successful in treating certain cases of PMS.

PHYSICAL AND EMOTIONAL SYMPTOMS

PMS sufferers, on average, eat four and a half times more dairy products than women who escape this syndrome. Saturated animal fat inhibits the formation of PGE1, an anti-inflammatory prostaglandin deficient in PMS sufferers. Evening primrose oil, blackcurrant or borage oil all enhance the production of PGE1. Vitamin E is also useful as an inhibitor against the formation of a PGE antagonist derived from the arachidonic acid found in animal products. The oils rich in gammalinoic acid need to be taken at a minimum dose of 1,500 mg every day of the month. A hypoglycaemic diet is ideal for PMS sufferers: it should be supplemented with evening primrose oil or any other oil high in GLA. Osteopathic adjustment may be necessary to relieve bloating and exercise certainly helps.

There are, in fact, not one but four different types of PMS. Women with PMS-A have abnormal hormone levels, too high in oestrogen and low in progesterone, and suffer from anxiety, irritability and nervous tension as a result. PMS-H women have water retention problems with subsequent bloating and breast pain. PMS-C women crave refined carbohydrates and feel weak and headachey. PMS-D women can get profoundly depressed, forgetful and confused. In their instance the progesterone is too high and oestrogen is too low. Women with PMS-A tend to eat large amounts of dairy produce, while those with PMS-H eat too much refined carbohydrates and those with PMS-C too much animal fat. PMS-Ds are especially vulnerable to the affects of environmental lead. All PMS sufferers are deficient in B complex and magnesium, both of which are closely involved with the mood altering chemicals in the brain. A magnesium deficiency is exacerbated by a diet high in dairy products, which also allows more lead to get into the body.

I have found that severe candida infections can exacerbate PMS, so it is worth getting this checked out.

Apart from following all the advice on a hypoglycaemic diet on page 179, take the following precrash tonic in the 10 days leading up to your period.

PRECRASH TONIC

Equal parts of:
chaste tree
wild yam
sarsaparilla
dandelion
valerian
uva ursi
corn silk
false unicorn
squawvine
blue cohosh
cramp bark
sage
ginger
blessed thistle.

Make as a tincture and take 30 drops four to five times a day in a little water. Once the period starts switch to Higher Nature's premens prevention (see Resource Directory). I found this an extremely successful formulation if followed faithfully over a period of some months.

FEMALE CORRECTIVE

This combination of herbs helps to rebuild a malfunctioning reproductive system and is an excellent general tonic. It nourishes the malfunctioning organs.
Equal parts of:
goldenseal root
blessed thistle
cayenne
cramp bark
false unicorn
ginger
red raspberry
squawvine
uva ursi.
Decoct and drink three cups a day.

PROSTATE GLAND PROBLEMS

Some 65% of men over 60 suffer from a prostate problem that it is entirely preventable.

A normal size prostate is about the size of a walnut but, when it becomes inflamed and swells, it puts pressure on the urethra and you may notice a deep, dull ache in the lower abdomen close to the rectum, get chronic backache or pain during ejaculation, see traces of blood in the urine or semen, or notice that it is taking longer than usual to empty the bladder. Any retained urine will cause cystitis, which in turn affects the kidneys and leads to a backlog of urinary waste in the bloodstream. A swollen prostate, if neglected, can become cancerous.

Avoid undue abstinence from sex and sexual intercourse without the natural conclusion of orgasm. Petting and withdrawal without orgasm will lead to a prolonged engorgement of the prostate gland and may result in functional and, occasionally, even structural damage. Walking is the best possible form of exercise for keeping the prostate gland healthy. Aim to walk for an hour a day.

The diet should be rich in raw seeds, especially pumpkin and sunflower seeds. These are high in protein and unsaturated fats and pumpkin seeds contain a male androgen hormone which is known to be beneficial to the prostate gland. Both seeds are also high in zinc and essential fatty acids and lack of these is known to be a contributing cause of prostate disorders. The diet should contain plenty of raw vegetables and fruits that are high in vitamin E and also wholewheat bread and wheatgerm as well as lecithin (available from health-food shops) and natural sources of vitamin D. Avoid coffee, alcohol and strong spices, which are known to be contributory causes of predisposition to prostatis.

When going to the toilet void all urine completely. Be careful not to strain but continue even if it takes a minute or longer until no more spurts can be obtained. By doing this bladder tone can be maintained.

The following exercise is a good way of keeping the prostate gland in good condition. Lie down on the floor flat on your back. Pull your knees up to your chest as far as possible then press the soles of both feet together. Maintaining this position lower the legs toward the floor as far as possible with a forceful movement. Repeat as many times as possible, up to 10.

The prostate also secretes hormones which are fed into the bloodstream and are a contributive factor to general health and well-being. So the herbal approach to this problem is necessarily two-pronged: one to help the hormone balance and the other to cleanse and maintain the bladder and kidneys and reduce the swelling.

RETAINED ENEMA

You can reduce the swelling by mixing together equal parts of cold-pressed safflower, olive and sesame oil, measuring out two tablespoons in all, and squeezing 10,000 IUs of oil based vitamin A and 1,000 IUs of vitamin E into the oil. Put the mixture into a small bulb syringe and squeeze it into the rectum just before bed, retaining it until your next bowel movement. Do this nightly, resting on the seventh day until the swelling is alleviated.

In addition to pumpkin seeds, which are rich in vitamins A, B, E and F, zinc, iron, phosphorus and calcium as well as a male androgen hormone (aim to eat at least a heaped handful of these daily), take 1,000 IUs of vitamin E daily working up to it gradually, and take another dose of A and D for one month only, 25,000 IUs of vitamin A and 1,000 IUs of vitamin D. Take two teaspoons of bee pollen daily, which is rich in natural oestrogens.

Avoid alcohol, spices and sugar absolutely and follow a clean vegan diet. Once a month you should do four or five days of internal cleansing on a fresh juice fast.

SITZ-BATHS

These are especially helpful in acute cases, relieving congestion in the pelvis and so helping with the pain. Use alternating hot and cold sitz-baths in either camomile or lemon balm. Sit in the hot bath for 15 minutes and the cold one for two to three minutes. If the pain is acute, use ice-cold retention enemas of well-strained camomile tea.

TONIC FOR PROSTATITIS

If the prostate becomes inflamed take the following mixture.
Equal parts of:
saw palmetto
sarsaparilla
Siberian ginseng
marshmallow root
chaparral
echinacea
goldenseal
Take 15 drops in tincture form five times a day in water as long as the infection lasts.

In addition to the tonic suggested, apply hot and cold packs to the prostate area, which is the area between the scrotum and the anus. Crushed ice wrapped in a face towel makes a simple ice pack. Apply the hot pack for four to eight minutes followed immediately with the cold pack for one to two minutes and do this routine two or three times over two sessions a day or more often if needed. This system of ice packs will reduce inflammation very quickly and give welcome relief.

Also make a pessary of equal parts of saw palmetto and echinacea root mixed in slippery elm and coconut butter inserting it in the anus before going to bed.

Check that there is no other infection in the body. I have on several occasions found heavy metal toxicity linked directly to prostatitis.

Last, but definitely not least, exercise the pubococcygeal muscle regularly by doing the Kegel exercises on page 182.

For general prostate maintenance Bioforce's Prostasan is excellent (see Resource Directory).

PSORIASIS

This very stubborn skin disease is characterized by the presence of red, scaly plaques on the arms and legs, particularly the elbows and knees, as well as the scalp and trunk. It affects 2% of the human race but is not contagious and in my experience intensive tar, sulphur or ultraviolet light treatment merely impede healing.

Naturopaths believe that the most common cause of psoriasis is a thinning of the walls of the small intestine, which allows poisons to enter the circulatory system and the lymph, thereby setting up irritations on the skin. This thinning may be the result of constipation, malabsorption of essential fatty acids, food allergy, improperly functioning kidneys or liver, previous immunizations or candidiasis. An iridology test is therefore imperative to enable the practitioner to adopt an appropriate approach.

Emotional factors must not be ignored: stress certainly makes the disease worse.

Treatment of psoriasis takes much time and perseverance for the best results although I did once put a patient on a 21-day grape fast and it cleared long-standing psoriasis up almost immediately, never to return. Generally I find the use of raw food coupled with lecithin supplementation particularly helpful together with zinc which is richly present in sunflower seeds, folic acid which is present in nutritional yeast and essential fatty acids. All animal products need to be strictly eliminated and prolonged supervised fasts ranging from one to three weeks are excellent if coupled with plenty of spirulina or chlorella and enemas or colonics. Indeed I have improved on Bernard Jensen's seven-day deep tissue cleansing programme which was specifically designed to heal psoriasis. This consists of fasting for seven consecutive days on organic vegetable juices with an emphasis on carrot juice, a colonic every day, some deep body work daily, regular hydrotherapy and plenty of outdoor exercise and natural light. Certainly sunbathing and sea water help to effect a temporary clearing and alternate hot and cold showers are useful. I advise a clean vegan diet and the application of a castor oil poultice to the abdomen six nights weekly, resting on the seventh.

To cleanse the colon and correct constipation use the formula on page 143 and check that the mid-thoracic area through to the sacral region in the spine is in alignment.

If regular sea bathing is not possible, take a homemade Epsom salt bath once a week (see page 47). The cider vinegar in it will help to restore acidity to the skin which is essential for restoration of health.

PYORRHOEA SEE GUM DISEASE

RHEUMATOID ARTHRITIS SEE ARTHRITIS AND RHEUMATISM

SCHIZOPHRENIA

The orthodox approach to schizophrenia includes tranquillizers and electro-convulsive therapy. Over the last 20 years, an accumulative body of research has pointed toward diet and nutrition as a central factor in schizophrenia, as well as some other mental illnesses. It seems the real causes of schizophrenia involve abnormal brain biochemistry due to a genetic or acquired condition involving one or more nutrients or, in some cases, toxins. However the average psychiatrist still refuses to believe that nutrition plays any part whatsoever in mental illness.

Hypoglycaemia is almost always involved in schizophrenia and may, in fact, be one of its most important contributing causes. Therefore, frequent small meals of high-quality natural food with an emphasis on slow-to-digest wholegrain products, plus an abundance of whole raw and sprouted seeds and nuts, is imperative. Almonds, sesame seeds, sunflower seeds and pumpkin seeds are particularly beneficial. A good quantity of high-quality protein is necessary but this should be of vegetable rather than animal origin. Soya beans, almonds, buckwheat, sesame seeds, sunflower seeds and all sprouted seeds, together with all vegetables and nutritional yeast, supply easily digestible proteins of good biological value and they are also rich in E and B vitamins as well as zinc and other trace minerals. This is particularly important. According to Dr Carl Pseiffer of the New Jersey Neuro-psychiatric Institute in Princeton, schizophrenia is primarily a biochemical disorder in the brain caused in general by mineral and trace element imbalances, particularly the deficiency of zinc combined with an excess of copper. Some 80% of the patients he worked with suffering from schizophrenia were found to have a deficiency of zinc and an excess of copper and iron in their body tissues. He prescribed high doses of zinc and manganese, which help to displace copper in the body and eliminate zinc deficiency and as a result claimed a 95% success rate.

In my own practice I found the best treatment of all for schizophrenia is repeated short juice fasts or, if the patient is able to manage it, a prolonged four- to six-week juice fast which normalizes all the body's functions and eliminates biochemical disorders and imbalances.

Such fasting should be undertaken only on expert advice and guidance from a practitioner conversant with this therapy and the patients should take juices or potassium broth at least every two hours.

Potassium broth maintains stable blood sugar levels. Overly sweet juices should be diluted half and half with filtered water.

It is also essential that supposed schizophrenics be checked for heavy metal poisoning which can produce schizophrenia-like symptoms. Cerebral allergies may also be a factor in schizophrenic behaviour. Faulty essential fatty acid metabolism or deficiency can be a contributing factor and in this instance flax seed oil can be very useful.

Because destructive self-condemnation can dog schizophrenics, sunshine, peace, quiet, kindness and love are essential. Meditation under supervision is also very helpful.

SCIATICA SEE BACK PAIN

Note: Potters make an excellent liquid extract remedy specifically for sciatica, which I have used with a great deal of success. Take two teaspoons in hot water every four hours (see Resources Directory). Acupuncture can also be particularly helpful for acute sciatic nerve pain.

SENILE DEMENTIA

This is commonly caused by poor circulation to the brain, resulting in cerebral atherosclerosis, prolonged nutritional deficiency, heavy metal overload, prolonged drug use and lack of exercise.

Prevention is much better than cure and far easier. The diet should consist of plenty of raw foods, the avoidance of heavy metals (from cooking in them or eating from tins), as well as aerobic exercise to maintain adequate circulation throughout the body. In addition to the diet and exercise regime recommended under heart disease, take 30 drops of *Ginkgo biloba* tincture four times a day or take the brain tonic.

BRAIN TONIC

> *Two parts of:*
> *ginkgo leaf*
> *gotu kola*
> *One part of:*
> *sweet flag root*
> *rosemary flowers*
> *sage leaf*
> *cayenne pepper*
> *European oak mistletoe*
>
> *Take 15 drops three times a day.*
> *Also do the slant-board exercises daily for 20 minutes (page 168) and take the seven times hot/cold head showers daily (page 50).*

SEPTICAEMIA

The treatment for septicaemia, or blood poisoning, is by herbal antibiotic, two or three every half hour.

Seek professional medical advice urgently.

SHINGLES

This is caused by the same virus that causes chickenpox in children and results in infection of the nerve fibres, characterized by the appearance of clusters of painful blisters wherever the branch of the affected nerves ends, most often on one side of the face or on the side of the trunk. You generally have to be very run down to get shingles so massive doses of vitamin C (stopping just short of diarrhoea) are particularly helpful.

REMEDY FOR SHINGLES

> *Two parts of:*
> *Echinacea*
> *goldenrod*
> *One part of:*
> *skullcap*
> *lobelia (only available from qualified medical herbalists)*
> *oats*
>
> *Take in tincture form 20 drops five or six times daily.*

Dab the affected area with equal parts of a tincture made from marigolds, lavender, goldenseal and myrrh, which will greatly relieve the itching.

If neuralgia persists after the blisters have cleared, treat this (see page 205).

SHOCK

I carry Dr Bach's Rescue Remedy, which consists of the tinctures of five different herbs, with me permanently and consider myself well equipped for an emergency with a bottle in my pocket. This deals with the emotional effects of shock which, if not helped immediately, can reverberate through the system for years, causing an insidious build-up of all sorts of psychological and physiological problems. When coupled with skullcap, it is one of the best remedies for short-term stress. (One size 0 capsule of the skullcap should be taken hourly as long as the acute crisis lasts.)

The Rescue Remedy should be diluted, four drops in 2 fl oz (50 ml) pure spring water to which add a little brandy or, if you are allergic to alcohol, cider vinegar as a preservative. Take four drops of the previously prepared mixture in one teaspoon (5 ml) water and hold it on the tongue for 30 seconds before swallowing. Repeat this at least four and up to six times daily. If the patient is unconscious, rub it into the lips or on the wrists. Rescue Remedy is available from some health food shops or by post (see Resources Directory).

Shock could be one of the main products of sudden and sometimes permanent cell changes in the body, and it is one of the major contributors in all disease, which is why I find the Rescue Remedy so invaluable. Have some on hand at all times. It comes in a tiny bottle with its own dropper and is easily slipped into a purse, pocket or the glove compartment of your car.

Alternatively, take one teaspoon of cayenne in hot water. In the event of a heart attack take three teaspoons of the powder or 30 drops of tincture of cayenne in a cup of water immediately and all at once. Then take 10 drops of tincture or half a teaspoon of cayenne in hot water every 15 minutes until normal colour returns.

....

Get medical help as quickly as possible.

....

SINUSITIS

Chronic sinusitis is generally the result of suppressing or failing to treat colds properly. Freshly squeezed grapefruit juice is particularly useful for clearing catarrh from the sinuses and after a three-day fast on this, follow a raw food diet. Check for heavy metal toxicity which in my experience has often been a contributing factor to sinusitis, and also check that the teeth and gums are in good order. Breathe in the vaporized oil from sage and hot water twice daily, keeping the eyes closed so that the steam doesn't sting. Rub fresh lemon juice externally over the sinuses or spray lemon juice and water as a douche with a nasal spray inside the nose. Nasal sprays are available from chemists.

SINUS TONIC

> *Equal parts of:*
> *freshly grated horseradish*
> *onion*
> *garlic*
> *ginger*
> *chili pepper.*
>
> *(The grating alone, by forcing you to breathe in the fumes, can be extremely effective.) Put this mixture in a wide-necked jar and cover with cider vinegar. Screw on a tight-fitting fitting lid and macerate for two weeks in an airing cupboard, shaking twice daily. Press the mixture out using if possible a wine press to extract every last drop and take two teaspoons before each meal.*

A poultice of grated onion on the back of the neck worn all night in bed and secured with a scarf is extremely helpful, as is a hot compress of plain water to the back of the neck and ice cubes on the forehead.

In acute cases Bioforce's SNS146, 25 drops on the tongue five times a day, is also very helpful (see Resources Directory).

SMOKING

You can live without food for several months, without water for up to five days, but without air, even if you have the lungs of Houdini, for about three minutes. Clean fresh air is the single most vital nutrient the body needs for its survival. I will not work with people who smoke (either tobacco or marijuana) unless they are willing to give it up. Here are some facts about smoking you may not already know.

- Cigarettes affect the circulatory system. The heart accelerates 20 to 25 beats per minute after one cigarette and so needs more oxygen, but the poisonous carbon monoxide from cigarettes actually forces oxygen out of the bloodstream.
- Cigarettes reduce blood flow to the hands and feet and it takes six hours after the last cigarette to get the blood flow back on an even keel. So if smoking is the first thing you do on rising and the last on sleeping, your circulation will probably only be normal for about two hours a day.
- Smoking depresses the immune system and this process takes three months to reverse once you have given up.
- Thinning of the bones is aggravated and may even be caused by smoking.
- Men who smoke get more problems with their prostate glands and women more severe menopausal problems.
- Smoking inhibits the functioning of the pancreas and may lead to hypogly-caemia.
- Smokers' ulcers heal more slowly than those of non-smokers, if at all.
- Tremors in the fingers increase by 39% after only one cigarette.
- If current trends persist, deaths from lung cancer in women will overtake deaths from breast cancer by the year 2000.
- Passive smoking greatly increases the risk of lung cancer, as well as heart disease, nasal sinus cancer and brain tumour. If you work an eight-hour day in the same room as someone who smokes 30 cigarettes a day you will have passively inhaled five cigarettes. This is enough, in the case of a pregnant woman, to affect the foetus.

COMPROMISES

If you simply cannot give up, try smoking your own mixture using herbs that do not contain nicotine. Coltsfoot is a tonic expectorant and actually decongests the tar-laden lungs, or try rosemary, mullein, yerba santa or sarsaparilla, spiced perhaps with cloves or cinnamon, mint, liquorice or even rose oil. A home-made smoking mixture (and there are some available in health-food stores ready made up) tastes nothing like tobacco but at least it is not physically addictive. It can be used as an in-between step to wean yourself off the habit of smoking altogether.

Lobelia, which contains lobeline, a substance similar to nicotine but without the same effect, reduces the sensation of need for nicotine but does not provide the effects that lead to addiction. Lobelia is on the poisons list and is only available from a medical herbalist.

Remember any burning plant material contains smoke and tar so herbal cigarettes should not be smoked except as a halfway step to stop smoking altogether.

AVERSION THERAPY

Every time you feel like a cigarette chew a piece of calamus root or dab some of the powdered herb on the tongue. If you smoke a cigarette after this it will make you physically sick.

Alternatively, restrict your smoking to an intensive one hour daily (enough to cause nausea in itself) and take 15 drops of lobelia tincture (available only from qualified medical herbalists) in water half an hour before this session and 15 minutes afterward. If you smoke more than one cigarette take 15 drops every 15 minutes after each cigarette. The result will be nausea or vomiting which mentally becomes enmeshed with smoking.

OTHER AIDS

- A two-week juice fast is helpful both to detoxify the body and overcome nicotine craving. Motivation for this, however, needs to be high.
- Coffee and tea need to be cut down to only three cups of each or both before attempting to give up.
- Stress levels can be reduced by plenty of exercise.
- Oral gratification by chewing a piece of liquorice root, provided the blood pressure is not dangerously high, is also helpful.
- A hypoglycaemic diet helps to smooth blood sugar curves and so strengthen willpower.
- Keep doses of vitamin C to just below diarrhoea level while giving up smoking. It is, among its many other assets, a good detoxifier and will help to combat the apathy and depression that may set in if willpower wavers.

MARIJUANA SMOKING

Even more damage is done to the lungs of marijuana smokers than heavy tobacco smokers. Its long-term effects can result in constant fatigue, an inability to study, poor memory retention, constant and recurrent illnesses, especially genital herpes, cold sores and skin problems, and lack of muscular co-ordination. It is also, of course, illegal to possess marijuana.

The cannabinoid substances in marijuana suppress the immune system and strongly interfere with vital cellular processes. The characteristic smell of cannabis smoke is enough to produce the same effects in a habitual marijuana smoker even when all the known active constituents have been removed – which means it is psychologically as well as physically addictive.

TO BEAT MARIJUANA

A good formula to help you get off it is:
Four parts of:
prickly ash
Two parts of:
ginseng
One part of:
bayberry bark
Icelandic moss

Put 4 oz (115 g) in 2 pts (1.1 litres) of water and stir well. Cover and macerate for two hours. Simmer for half an hour then strain. Add one cup of blackstrap molasses and one cup of glycerine to the liquid and dissolve over heat while stirring. Cool, bottle and take three tablespoons four times daily between meals, the last dose to be taken just before bed.

SPASTIC COLON SEE IRRITABLE BOWEL SYNDROME

SPRAINS

No matter which joint is sprained, apply an ice pack to the area immediately. A packet of frozen peas will do in an emergency, while you prepare a proper ice pack by crushing ice with a rolling pin in a plastic bag before transferring it into a pillowcase. Alternatively, soak a hand towel in cold water, wring it out till it stops dripping and place it folded on foil in the freezer. Let it stay there until crystals form but the towel is not frozen solid. This follows the contours of the injured area.

If massaging an area with ice on a regular basis (and this has been found to be very useful in 80% of patients suffering from chronic pain of various types, ranging from lower back pain, rheumatoid and osteoarthritis and cancer, supplying relief for up to three hours), fill a polystyrene or plastic cup with water, freeze it, then peel the cup to below ice level. You then have a block of ice and a cold-resistant handle. Keep the ice moving to avoid skin damage and stop the treatment the moment skin numbness occurs.

When treating a sprain secure the ice pack close to the body by wrapping round firmly in more plastic and refresh as needed. Leave this on for 30 minutes, elevating the joint to stop effusion. If the fingers and toes turn blue you have overdone it. Loosen the plastic bandage in this instance and gently rub the blue areas to restore circulation, then apply a generous layer of the following trauma oil: equal parts of St John's wort, marigold and arnica macerated in olive oil. Keep massaging the area with this mixture as often as possible and take as little exercise as possible. If necessary apply a sling to immobilize a sprained shoulder or enforce complete bed rest to heal back sprain.

If in any doubt at all whether the joint may be fractured, seek immediate medical help.

STOMACH ULCER SEE DUODENAL ULCER
STRESS SEE ANXIETY
STYES

Always ensure that the bowels are working properly and bathe the eyes with freshly made and meticulously strained decoction of equal parts of eyebright, burdock and sarsaparilla. Take one cup of the mixture internally three times a day with meals.

If the stye is unbearably itchy, rub it with a piece of raw potato or dab on tincture of goldenseal which may sting a bit but which proves very effective.

SUNBURN

If severe, essential oil of lavender applied on a dampened piece of gauze or muslin and left on as a poultice is very effective. This should be repeated every four hours. If less severe apply the cooling aloe vera gel available from Xxynergy (see Resources Directory).

Remember that prevention is always better than cure. Protect yourself with a sunscreen with a sufficiently high SPF.

SWOLLEN GLANDS

Wherever there are lymph glands in the body they can become swollen. These congregate in the groin, behind the knees, in the throat and in the armpits and signal that a distressed lymph system is no longer able to cope. Embark on a three-day fruit juice fast followed by a raw food diet to cleanse the lymph system. Dry skin brush daily (see page 87) followed by hot and cold showers (see page 51). If you can find one, have manual lymphatic drainage done by a therapist qualified in this area. Ensure you are not constipated. When well enough take up some form of exercise that will help pump lymph effectively around the body. Trampolining is best but consider skipping or swimming if this is not practical.

FORMULA FOR HEALTHY LYMPH GLANDS

Dr Christopher and I have used the following formulation successfully many times. Three parts of:
mullein
One part of:
lobelia (only available from qualified herbalists).

Make an infusion and drink half a cup three times a day until the glands are back to normal. Save the residual herbs for a poultice and apply as warm as possible to the swollen area before bed leaving it on all night. Alternatively, apply a hot compress of the tea to the area as above.

TEETHING AND TOOTHACHE

Rubbing gums with a little honey and a tiny pinch of salt may take away some of the pain of teething, but generally you will find you need stronger measures. If a child is able to chew without swallowing, give him or her a piece of arrowroot, liquorice or marshmallow root to chew on. Also make up a slippery elm poultice turning it into a paste with a double decoction of camomile. Pack this to the sore gum. It doesn't matter if this is swallowed.

DIARRHOEA WHILE TEETHING

Mix equal parts of anise, caraway, dill and fennel. Pound as finely as possible with a pestle and mortar and add enough slippery elm to mix to a poultice consistency with hot water spreading the whole mixture over the stomach. Give only weak yarrow tea, ½ oz (15 g) to 1 pt (575 ml), four teaspoons every 20 minutes, until the worst of the diarrhoea has subsided. If the diarrhoea doesn't calm down fairly quickly, feed the child slippery elm gruel by the teaspoon.

Persistent diarrhoea in a baby needs medical attention.

ACCIDENTS WITH TEETH

These often look horrendous and are more upsetting for the parent than the child. If the trauma is very severe, either breaking or loosening the tooth, the blood and nerve supplies may be severed which means that the tooth becomes dead. Such a tooth will become infected after varying amounts of time. Signs of infection include pain, unusual mobility or looseness of the tooth, or a whitehead on the outside of the gum. However, after any accident a tooth can be darkened and become discoloured which is simply the result of blood entering the inner pulp of the tooth. This does not necessarily mean that the tooth is dead.

Call a dentist in the case of a dental accident and book an emergency consultation. If the tooth is still in the socket but severely displaced the dentist may be able to realign it as long as the child is brought in for a consultation immediately after the accident. If there are signs of infection, the dentist may want to do root canal work, cap the tooth or remove it altogether.

Initially, if there is active bleeding the person offering treatment should press a tissue directly over the area hard until the bleeding stops. Ice can be applied if it makes the recipient more comfortable. If the tooth is knocked out or cracked, moves freely or the gum is swollen or bleeding phone the dentist immediately. Dr Bach's Rescue Remedy is invaluable here to alleviate shock (see Resources Directory). A tooth that has been knocked out should be placed under the tongue while you get to the dentist, in case he or she can replace it.

TOOTHACHE

First try using dental floss between the aching tooth and its neighbours because impacted food may have set up the pain. If this does not work, make an appointment with your dentist. In the meantime, apply an ice pack against the jaw on the infected side and if this makes things worse apply a hot water bottle.

If you see a cavity make sure it is clean (sterile cotton on the end of a toothpick helps here) then pack into the hole a piece of cotton cloth saturated with oil of cloves or garlic. Rub the surrounding gum with tincture of cayenne (or if this is unbearable oil of cloves) and repeat as necessary. Also rub ice over the web of skin between the thumb and index finger on the same side of the body as the pain is. This is the acupressure point used to relieve toothache.

THRUSH SEE CANDIDIASIS

THYROID DISORDER SEE GOITRE

TONSILLITIS

If tonsillitis is chronic, investigate whether there is a problem of allergy or nutritional deficiency particularly of the B complex, vitamin C, zinc and iron. A diet with too many dairy products, sugar and starches and a deficiency of green vegetables will lead to acidity, toxicity and catarrh throughout the body. Spinal lesions in the neck may reduce blood and lymph flow to the tonsils and adenoids so osteopathic intervention may be necessary. Removing the tonsils will not make the problem go away; tonsils are a valuable lymph aggregate and if they swell this is an early warning sign that should not be ignored.

TEA FOR TONSILLITIS

As long as the patient can swallow, administer one cup of the following herbal tea, proportionate to age, six times a day.

Two parts of:
echinacea
red sage
One part of:
goldenseal
calendula.

Gargle with a teaspoon of goldenseal tincture or a teaspoon of myrrh in a cup of water as often as needed. Spraying neat tincture of echinacea directly on to the glands using a hand spray obtainable from chemists is very helpful both for the infection and for the pain. An external compress as for swollen glands is very helpful (see page 225). Ice cream is commonly given for tonsillitis but this is one of the worst things you can do, in view of its mucus-forming potential. The best is to fast on juices until the infection is cleared.

TRAVEL SICKNESS

Astronauts are given ginger to stop sickness in space. To relieve travel sickness, take a wine glass of hot fresh ginger tea or two size 0 capsules of powdered ginger as often as needed. This has been proved to be twice as effective as Dramamine.

A particularly effective cure for seasickness is 3 drops of essential oil of marjoram in a little honey water.

Pressure on an acupuncture point called *nei-kuan* helps relieve seasickness or travel sickness. This point is on the surface of the inside of both forearms, three finger widths away from the crease of the wrist and in the centre between the two flex tendons. Press this point with the tip of the thumb (short fingernails help here). Repeat as often as necessary. Seabands, specially designed wrist straps with a rounded plastic button that will do this for you, are available from chemists, and neck pads that apply light pressure to appropriate pressure points in the neck are increasingly available.

It helps to focus on distant objects rather than on fast-moving nearby ones while travelling in a car or train. Ensure children, while safely strapped in, are elevated enough to see out of the window. On a plane sit on a seat over the wheels rather than in the tail which moves more than the rest of the plane. On a ship stay on deck as much as you can and keep busy.

VARICOSE VEINS

A family history of low arterial blood pressure makes a person more liable to varicosity. Nearly 10% of pregnant women get varicose veins during the course of their pregnancy. Veins in the legs are particularly prone. The problem is exacerbated by calcium deficiency, by standing for long periods, which impedes the circulation, and by wearing constrictive clothing or shoes. A decoction of oak bark tea is very helpful. Soak cotton or silk stockings in it and pull these over the legs at night wrapping round with plastic to prevent leaks.

Bioforce's Hyperisan tincture taken internally is also helpful (see Resources Directory).

WARTS

There are all sorts of ways to remove warts and you may need to try more than one.

- Apply a generous poultice of castor oil over the wart every morning and night for several months.
- Apply the juice squeezed out of fresh celandine directly on to the warts.
- Apply the milky juice of fresh, barely ripe figs directly on to the warts.
- Cut a raw potato and rub it on several times a day.
- Eat four tablespoons of asparagus purée twice a day.
- Apply the milky juice squeezed out of dandelion leaves several times a day.
- Apply a slice of raw garlic adhered over the wart with stretchy sticking plaster every night.

The patient's faith in the treatment often plays the most important role in achieving results. This seems to be particularly true as far as warts are concerned.

WATER RETENTION

This is common as part of premenstrual tension just before a period but can happen at any time due to levels of certain hormones in the body. The commonest symptoms are breast tenderness, swollen abdomen, headaches, constipation, irritability and swelling in the ankles, feet, hands or face. To test for water retention, or oedema, press the thumb against the shin bone for 20 seconds and if, after removing it, a white indented area is noticed which fails to fill up within five seconds and return to its normal colouring, there is definite water retention. In this case it may take up to two minutes for the white area in the indentation to normalize.

One of the safest ways to treat this is by drinking dandelion root coffee. Unlike medical diuretics, this will not leach potassium from the system. Cut out all forms of salt from the diet including hidden salt in processed food; those foods that are rich in vitamin C increase urine flow which helps to alleviate symptoms. The kidney tea and the kidney tonic on page 85 is also an excellent and safe diuretic.

WHOOPING COUGH SEE CHILDHOOD DISEASES

WORMS

Worms outrank even cancer as the human race's deadliest enemy. According to the World Health Organisation every fourth person is infected by worms; if tropical worms, including hook- and whipworms, are included, possibly every third member of the human race has intestinal parasites.

These parasites range in size from microscopic single-celled creatures to 24 ft (7.3 m) tapeworms. Some of my patients, during the course of a thorough bowel clean, are quite stunned to see worms come out, since they have never displayed the usual symptoms, of anal irritation, dry lips during the day and wet at night, a little pool of spit dribbled on to the pillow at night, loss of appetite, irritability, dark circles under the eyes, frequent colds, anaemia, sudden loss of weight, weakness and lassitude.

As well as tapeworms, roundworms and threadworms, there are also hook worms, all floating around in a variety of unpleasant places, eager to crawl into a comfortable and nourishing body. You can ingest them by eating unwashed foods that have been grown on soil fertilized with manure that has not been properly composted. Soil in China and parts of the Third World is fertilized with human excreta; when having a colonic irrigation after returning from a trip to China, I was not unduly surprised to witness two quite large worms beating a hasty retreat from my colon. These were in fact roundworms. Such worms if left to breed (and a single female produces about 200,000 eggs each day) may become entangled in the intestines, blocking various organs and ducts.

In order to avoid them:

- always wash your hands after going to the toilet
- do not eat anything which has been composted in human faeces
- always wash all vegetables
- do not allow cats to lick the face or hands: field mice can be infected by excrement from dogs and this in turn can be transmitted to cats and from these to humans.

The larvae of *Echinococcus* can form small blister-like swellings in the human liver, as well as attacking the intestine, so do not allow cats who are infested with worms to sleep on the bed.

Tapeworms are acquired from poorly prepared pork and from uncooked fish. They are the most difficult worms to get rid of and linger in the colon, slightly lowering iron absorption year by year but rarely going far enough to be fatal (obviously no parasite will actually kill its host – that would be self-defeating). Tapeworms can induce a particularly severe form of anaemia.

Hookworms tend to occur in tropical countries and are contracted by people walking barefooted in areas where faeces have been excreted from pigs, dogs, cattle and humans. As with tapeworms, hookworms primarily cause anaemia but they can also lead to respiratory problems, nausea and diarrhoea.

Threadworms are the most common worm infestation and one in five British schoolchildren is infected with them at some time or another. They are spread by inhaling or ingesting the eggs and the female creeps out of the anus at night to lay her eggs externally. If the anus is then scratched the eggs lodge under the fingernails and can be passed on. A single female is capable of laying 10,000 eggs which can mature in two weeks. They can produce symptoms which appear to be like appendicitis. As with all other parasitic infestations threadworms develop best if the vitality is low and the diet is poor, particularly if it is rich in refined carbohydrates and sugar and low in fibre. If someone in the family has threadworms, hygiene is obviously of the essence and all underwear, sheets and towels need to be boiled.

TREATMENT

Worms revel in a constipated colon and enjoy sugar and acid conditions. So a high-fibre, alkaline and sugar-free diet is the best means of prevention and cure. Foods which worms particularly dislike include garlic, onions, pomegranates, pumpkin seeds, cabbage, pawpaw, horseradish, figs and pineapple.

Dr Shook, my teacher's teacher, advises the following regime to get rid of both tapeworms and roundworms. Begin by eating all the foods that worms hate (together with other foods, of course) and drink a strong cup of wormwood tea in the morning and at night for three days using the usual proportions for an infusion. On the fourth day take a cup of senna tea to cleanse the bowel of the dead parasites. Add some liquorice to the tea to prevent griping pains (any other anthelmintic may be used instead of wormwood if it seems more appropriate; these include aloe, butternut, elecampane, hyssop and wormseed). Wormwood tastes very bitter and it works just as effectively in pill form. Pomegranate seeds are a tastier and more palatable alternative.

To assist tapeworm evacuation, sit on a bucket with some warm milk in it when it is time to empty the bowel. Cold air stops the tapeworm from leaving, the warm air entices it out. It is vital to ensure that the head with its digestive suckers, which look like two big eyes, emerges so inspect the contents of the bucket afterward.

Threadworms need to be treated with garlic enemas or a peeled clove of garlic with the inner skin left unbroken inserted directly into the anus at night. Rub garlic oil externally around the anus. Quassia tea made as a decoction in equal parts with liquorice should be taken internally, two teaspoons before meals three times a day.

Because the removal of worms is a tricky business, you are advised to seek the professional help of a qualified medical herbalist conversant in these matters.

WOUNDS, MINOR CUTS AND BRUISES

Place the wound in ice-cold water to stop the bleeding and reduce inflammation; alternatively apply cayenne pepper directly externally. Ensure the cut is absolutely clean; proper cleansing is vital to help the wound heal easily and to prevent infection. If after a day or two the cut becomes tender and begins to swell or redden, indicating that it has become infected, there is a very simple remedy. If the infection is mild, soak the injured area in warm water for 15 minutes, two or three times a day. The warmth of the water increases blood flow which brings antibodies and white blood cells to the area. Tea-tree or thyme oil applied directly to the wound will sting but will certainly stop infection. A poultice of powdered comfrey root will accelerate the healing – if the cut is very superficial use comfrey ointment.

Apply neat cayenne pepper over bleeding cuts; this sounds radical, and it certainly stings, but it works.

If a person cuts off a large flap of skin, such as a finger tip, pressure should be applied to the cut to stop the bleeding. The piece of skin should be put into ice-cold water or salt water – half a teaspoon of salt to 2 pints (1.1 litres) of water – and taken along to the doctor. Generally it is possible to stitch the flap back on.

If the bleeding is copious and difficult to stop, take a quarter of a teaspoon of cayenne in water, preferably warm, internally and apply a tourniquet externally. This is best applied by somebody properly trained in first aid: improper use can result in blood vessel and nerve damage. However the majority of cuts are minimal and rapidly heal by themselves. A cut needs the attention by a doctor only if it is deep or doesn't stop bleeding readily or contains dirt or foreign bodies that cannot be easily extracted. You may consider a cut deep enough if it goes through the skin and is long enough so that the sides of the cut separate and do not stay together. When a cut is this deep shiny connective tissues or yellow globules of fat can be seen in the wound.

Whereas scrapes and minor cuts seem to be part and parcel of early childhood, puncture wounds and many lacerations can be prevented. Children should be instructed at a very early age of the dangers and proper use of sharp objects like scissors, knives and tools. Puncture wounds are most commonly caused by nails in boards so any such boards with nails or tacks sticking out or sharp scraps of metal should obviously be removed from areas where children play. Large scrapes are generally caused by falls on cement or gravel when children are running or riding bikes; obviously parents should supervise children when engaged in such play.

YEAST INFECTION SEE CANDIDIASIS

RESOURCES DIRECTORY

ESSENTIAL OILS

DANIELE RYMAN'S ESSENTIAL OILS

Can be purchased through mail order by writing to her at Daniele Ryman Clinic, Park Lane Hotel, Piccadilly, London W1Y 8BX. Telephone 0171 753 6708.

BUTTERBUR & SAGE

7 Tessa Road, Reading, Berkshire RG1 8HH
Telephone 0118 9505100 Fax 0118 9576300
I have not encountered commercially available essential oils made to the high standards of this company. Most experienced aromatherapists agree with me.

ENVIRONMENTAL PRODUCTS

MOUNTAIN BREEZE IONIZER

6 Priors Wood Place, Skelmersdale, Lancashire WN8 9QB
Telephone 01695 21155

FOLIAGE FOR CLEAN AIR COUNCIL

Telephone 001 703534 5268

WHOLISTIC [SIC] RESEARCH COMPANY

Brighthaven, Robin's Lane, Lolworth, Cambridge CB3 8HH
Telephone 01954 781074
Particularly knowledgeable about ELF reduction and VDUs; supplies daylight simulation light bulbs and other useful information about SAD syndrome, including contacts for equipment. Supplier of douche and enema kits. The company also supplies Philips Daylight Blue and Sungrolite light bulbs, both of which provide light which more closely resembles daylight, enhancing visual accuracy and making reading easier. Philips Daylight Blue bulbs are also readily available from most electrical shops. The company also supplies wheatgrass juice presses and reverse-osmosis water filters.

DIAGNOSTIC TESTS

KEN ANDREWS

59 Telford Crescent, Leigh, Lancs WN7 5LY
Telephone 01942 678092
Supplies a list of vega testers.

JOHN MORLEY

140 Harley Street, London NW1 1AH
Telephone 0171 487 2617
Supplies mercury testing and vega tests.

JACK LEVENSON

1 Welby House, 62 Welbey Street, London W1N 7SB
Telephone 0171 486 3127
UK leader in mercury testing.

HIGHER NATURE LIMITED

The Nutrition Centre, Burwash Common, East Sussex TN19 7LX
Telephone 01435 882880
For osteoporosis checking.

BIOLAB

The Stonehouse, 9 Weymouth Street, London W1M 3FF
Telephone 0171 636 5959
Tests for *Candida albicans*, parasites and blood disorders.

HOME KITS

KITTY CAMPION

25 Curzon Street, Basford, Newcastle-under-Lyme, Staffordshire ST5 0PD
Telephone 01782 711592 Fax 01782 713274
Supplier of tea-tree pessaries, skin brushes, douche and enema kits and most of the composite herbal formulae mentioned in this book. Also supplier of Nature's Superfoods which contains most of the ingredients mentioned on p 18, as well as deep heat oil and trauma oil, and can offer colonic irrigation. She has also trained many colonic irrigationists in the country.

COLGATE MEDICAL LIMITED

1 Fairacres Estate, Dedworth Road, Windsor, Berkshire SL4 4LE
Telephone 01753 860378
Supplies Femina Cones, for testing and strengthening pelvic-floor muscles (Kegel muscles).

XXYNERGY

Lower Elsted, Midhurst, West Sussex GU29 0JT
Telephone 01730 813642
Supplies spirulina and biogenic aloe vera juice, as well as aloe vera gel for sunburn.

EARTHRISE

All Seasons Healthcare, Southsea, Hants PO15 1PL
Telephone 01705 755660
Supplies spirulina and biogenic aloe vera juice, as well as aloe vera gel for sunburn.

SAVANT DISTRIBUTION LTD

7 Wayland Croft, Adel, Leeds L516 8LX
Telephone 0113 2301993
Advice and an excellent blend of organic sunflower, safflower and flax seed oil.

HIGHER NATURE LIMITED

The Nutrition Centre, Burwash Common, East Sussex TN19 7LX
Telephone 01435 882880
All their formulations come in vegetarian capsules and they supply flax seed oil in bottled form. They also supply a transdermal cream, Pro-gen, made of wild yam, which is an excellent alternative to HRT.

H.H.C. LIMITED

67A Beech Hill, Hadley Wood, Barnet, Herts EN4 0JW
Telephone 0181 441 8352 Fax 0181 441 9950
Supplier of Vision Essentials.

VITA NATURA

PO Box 67F, Chessington, Surrey, KT9 1YL
Supplies Veggi-Wash, a pesticide cleanser for vegetables.

FOOD SAFE

Northampton NN6 7PD
Telephone 01788 510415
Sells a pesticide cleanser for vegetables.

RESIDENTIAL AND NON-RESIDENTIAL WORKSHOPS

THE BRISTOL CANCER HEALTH CENTRE

Grove House, Cornwallis Grove, Clifton, Bristol BS8 4PG
Telephone 01272 743216
Offers residential tuition courses to combat cancer.

KITTY CAMPION

Runs residential natural healing workshops in the UK and Europe throughout the year. She also offers home tuition by videos and home-study workbooks.

THE BRITISH SOCIETY FOR NUTRITIONAL MEDICINE

5 Somerhill Road, Hove, East Sussex BN3 1RP
This society is interested in the effects of food on health.

ASSOCIATIONS

ALCOHOLICS ANONYMOUS

Head Office
11 Redcliffe Gardens, London SW10 9BQ
Telephone 0171 352 9779

ALCOHOLICS ANONYMOUS

61 Great Dover Street, London SE1 4YF
Telephone 0171 403 0888
For the families of alcoholics.

ACTION ON SMOKING AND HEALTH (ASH)

5–11 Mortimer Street, London W1H 9PL
Telephone 0171 224 0743
Publishes information leaflets and advice on how to give up.

MYALGIC ENCEPHALOMYELITIS

The Moss, Third Avenue, Stanford-le-Hope, Essex SS17 8EL
Telephone 01375 642466
An organization to help sufferers of ME.

NATIONAL CHILDBIRTH TRUST

9 Queensborough Terrace, London W2
Telephone 0171 221 3833
An organization interested in empowering women to have the type of delivery they would like, and offering help and support to breastfeeding mothers.

NATIONAL PURE WATER ASSOCIATION

Bank Farm, Aston Pigott, Westbury, Shrewsbury ST5 9HH
Telephone 01784 383 445
This organization is interested in the quality of water and sends out regular newsletters.

EAST MERE MARKETING

2A Chequers Court, Huntingdon, Cambs PE18 6LJ
Telephone 01480 455588
Provides water filtration systems.

SCHIZOPHRENIA ASSOCIATION OF GREAT BRITAIN

Bryn Hyfryd, The Crescent, Bangor, Gwynedd LL57 2AG
Telephone 01248 354048
An organization to help sufferers from schizophrenia.

THE SOIL ASSOCIATION

86–88 Colston Street, Bristol BF1 5BB
Telephone 0117 290661
Vouchsafes for the safety of organic produce.

THE VEGETARIAN SOCIETY

Parkdale, Dunham Road, Altrincham, Cheshire WA14 4QG
Telephone 0161 928 0793

VEGAN SOCIETY

7 Battle Road, St Leonards on Sea, East Sussex TN37 7AA
Telephone 01424 427393

VIVA

12 Queens Square, Brighton, East Sussex BN1 3FD
Telephone 01273 777688
Promotes vegan and vegetarian lifestyles; sells an excellent video tape called *A Diet for All Reasons* by Dr Clapper. Enclose an SAE for information.

MANUAL LYMPHATIC DRAINAGE ASSOCIATION

8 Wittenham Lane, Dorchester on Thames, Oxon OX10 7JW
Telephone 01865 340385

THE EUROPEAN HERBAL PRACTITIONERS ASSOCIATION

Offers guidance on qualified herbal practitioners trained by Kitty Campion or with the National Institute of Herbal Medicine, or the General Council and Register of Consultant Medical Herbalists. Write to Kitty Campion; SAE appreciated.

NATURAL MEDICINE SOCIETY

Edith Lewis House, Back Lane, Ilkeston, Derby DE7 8EJ

ENVIRONMENTAL AIDS

NATURAL SOCIETY FOR CLEAN AIR

136 North Street, Brighton, East Sussex BN1 1RG
Telephone 01273 26313
An organization interested in the quality of air.

PROPOLIS

The New Zealand Natural Food Company Limited
9 Holt Close, Highgate Wood, London N10 3HW
Telephone 0181 444 5660

COMMUNITY FOODS LIMITED

Micross, Brent Terrace, London NW2 1LT
Telephone 0181 208 2966
Supplies natural sanitary towels.

BACH FLOWER REMEDIES

Available from homeopathic chemists and health-food stores throughout the country as well as from:

DR EDWARD BACH CENTRE

Mount Vernon, Sotwell, Wallingford, Oxfordshire OX10 0PZ
Telephone 01491 834678

HERBAL SUPPLIERS

THE HERBAL APOTHECARY

103 The High Street, Syston, Leicester LE7 1BQ
Telephone 0116 602690
Also suppliers of powdered herbs and gelatine capsules. Please note: before ordering capsules specify if you require vegetarian ones in bulk, i.e. not less than 1lb (½ kg) at a time.

SOLGAR VITAMINS LIMITED

Solgar House, Chiltern Centre, Asheridge Road, Chesham, Buckinghamshire HP5 2PY
This company supplies Earth Source, a good combination of many of the Superfoods, together with single herbs and combination formulas which are grown and processed to an extremely high standard; mainly packed in vegetarian capsules.

BLACKMORES LIMITED

Unit 7, Poyle Tech Centre, Willow Road, Poyle, Colnbrook, Buckinghamshire SL3 0PD
This is a long-established Australian company which uses organic herbs only, grown, harvested and processed to very high standards. What I particularly like about them is that they donate part of their turnover to environmental causes all over the world and are acutely aware of the strain on certain herbal resources worldwide, choosing instead to use alternatives wherever possible in any new formulae, rather than strain existing dwindling crops. They also have a very strict cruelty-free policy.

BIOFORCE UK LIMITED

Olympic Business Park, Dundonald, Ayrshire KA2 9BE
Telephone 01563 851177

I have dealt with this company for many years and admire the fact that, uniquely among herbal manufacturers, they use only freshly harvested herbs in their tinctures. The herbs are cultivated in a remote north-eastern corner of Switzerland between 800 and 1500 ft (250 and 460 m) above sea level which encourages the condensation of the healing properties in them. This company is also particularly strict about harvesting protocols. For example, *Echinacea purpurea* is harvested when it reaches 3 to 4 ft (0.9 to 1.2 m) in height when 50% of the flowers are in bloom and 50% in bud. Harvesting takes place after midday.

While many professional herbalists in practice, including myself, are particularly keen to harvest their own herbs freshly whenever possible, most commercially available herbal tinctures are not manufactured to Bioforce's particularly high standards. All Bioforce's products are readily available in health-care shops.

BIOCARE LIMITED

54 Northfield Road, Kings Norton, Birmingham B30 1JH
Telephone 0121 433 3727

This company is run by a team of extremely experienced chemists and its unique formulations are highly innovatory and of a very high standard. Biocare's products are available direct from the company and through herbal practitioners.

XXYNERGY HEALTH PRODUCTS

Lower Elsted, Midhurst, West Sussex GU29 9JT

This company imports extremely high-quality spirulina from the clean waters around New Zealand, so I particularly condone the purity and excellence of its product. They are suppliers of biogenic aloe vera juice which is organically grown and prepared in a unique way which does not denature or destroy its delicate enzymes and vital biogenic stimulators. I know of no comparable aloe vera juice.

MARIGOLD HEALTH FOODS LIMITED

Unit 10, St Pancras Commercial Centre, London NW1 0BY
Telephone 0171 267 7368

This company sells superb nutritional yeast flakes under the brand name Engevita. They also supply the House of Mistry's natural soap to health-food outlets.

A. NELSON & COMPANY LIMITED

5 Endeavour Way, Wimbledon, London SW19 9UE
Telephone 0181 946 8527
Makes a superb range of herbal ointments and creams. I particularly like this company because, like Bioforce, they use as many fresh base herbs as they can. Scientific testing using chromatography proves that fresh herbal preparations contain more of the active constituents and are more stable than their counterparts made from dried herbs.

POTTERS

Leyland Mill Lane, Wigan, Lancashire WN1 2SB
Telephone 01942 34761
This company makes an excellent range of herbal syrups for coughs and colds, as well as herbal tonics.

NEAL'S YARD APOTHECARY

2 Neal's Yard, Covent Garden, London WC2 9DP
Telephone 0171 379 7662

BALDWIN'S

173 Walworth Road, London SE17 1RW
Telephone 0171 703 5550
Both Neal's Yard and Baldwin's supply small quantities of herbs by post.

D. NAPIER & SONS

18 Bristol Place, Edinburgh, Scotland EH1 1EZ
Telephone 0131 225 5542

EDGAR CAYCE CENTRE

13 Prospect Terrace, New Kyo, Stanley, Co Durham DH9 7TF
Telephone 01207 237696
Sells cold-pressed castor oil and pure woollen flannel poultices.

MERCURY FREE DENTISTRY
HESHAM EL-ESSAWY

121 Harley Street, London W1N 1DH
Telephone 0171 935 3960

JACK LEVENSON

1 Welbeck House, 62 Welbeck Street, London W1N 7SB
Telephone 0171 486 3127
SAE appreciated

JOHN ROBERTS B.CH.D

141 Whitworth Road, Rochdale, Lancashire OL12 0RE
Telephone 01706 525905

also at:

10A Ashfield Road, Cheadle, Cheshire SK8 1BB

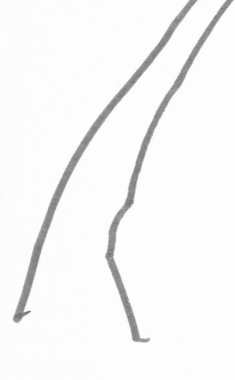

MEDICAL GLOSSARY

agoraphobia	fear of open spaces
allergen	a substance which provokes an allergic response
allopathic	meaning treatment by a conventional medicine, as practised by a graduate of a medical school
amenorrhoea	lack of menstruation
anaemia	lack of haemoglobin in the blood
angina pectoris	heart disease manifested by chest pain or exertion
anorexia	self-starvation
anxiety	nervous disorder characterized by a state of excessive uneasiness
bartholin cysts	cysts which form as a result of the infection of the bartholin glands (situated outside the vaginal opening)
bulimia	condition characterized by eating and vomiting cycles
cancer	malignant growths which invade healthy tissue and destroy it, often spreading to other parts of the body unchecked by the immune system
Candida albicans	a fungal infection which commonly affects the vagina, but may also affect other areas (such as the inside of the mouth or intestine)
cervical erosion	where the cells which normally occur in the inner lining of the cervix appear on the outside, causing redness, excessive production of mucus and sometimes bleeding
chilblains	itchy, red swelling caused by impaired blood supply and poor circulation
chlamydia	trachomatic micro-organisms which can affect cells in the cervix, bladder and Fallopian tubes
claustrophobia	dread of confined spaces
colitis	inflammation of the colon
constipation	infrequent bowel movements
cystitis	bacterial infection of the bladder
delirium tremens (DTs)	violent delirium characterized by tremors and hallucinations caused by coming off high alcohol intake abruptly

depression	mental illness
diarrhoea	where the colon becomes irritated and goes into overdrive
dioxin	one of a group of chemicals that are among the most toxic known, often used in defoliant weedkillers
diverticulitis	weakness in the colon wall causing the development of infected pouches (diverticula)
dysmenorrhoea	difficult and painful menstruation
dyspepsia	indigestion
dysplasia	abnormality of growth, at any level from the cell to the whole organ; abnormalities may include the size, shape and rate of multiplication of cells
endometriosis	tissue which normally lines the uterus found in other parts of the body
emmenagogue	a substance that promotes normal menstruation
fibroids	hard, lumpy, non-malignant growths of smooth muscle and fibrous connective tissue
genital warts	viral infection of the genital area
haemorrhoids	engorged veins inside or outside the anus
hiccups	involuntary spasms of the diaphragm and vocal cords
homeopathy	a system of medicine in which patients are treated with a highly diluted dose of a medicine which, in a healthy person, would result in the symptoms which are being treated
hyperactivity	abnormally high activity (usually found in children)
hypertension	high blood pressure
hyperventilation	overbreathing
hypoglycaemia	low blood sugar
iatrogenic	meaning 'physically produced', this is applied to the side-effects of a medical treatment, such as drowsiness caused by some cough medicine, or the hair loss that results from chemotherapy
incontinence	inability to retain urine
indigestion	burning pain or discomfort on eating
insomnia	inability to sleep
iridology	a diagnostic system based on the belief that the iris offers information on the state of the body
irritable bowel syndrome	nervous spasmodic colon
kidney stones	calcareous growths in the kidneys
leaky gut syndrome	increased gut permeability
leucorrhoea	excessive white vaginal discharge

lipoprotein	a spherical protein found in the blood stream which carries fats and cholesterol around the body; high-density lipoproteins contain a lot of protein and a little fat and carry cholesterol from tissues to the liver; low-density lipoproteins contain a little protein and a great deal of cholesterol and carry it to the arteries; LDLs are considered as 'bad': HDLs as 'good'
metrorrhagia	uterine haemorrhage outside of normal menstruation, recurrent headaches with visual and/or gastrointestinal disturbance
migraine	recurrent headaches with visual and/or gastro-intestinal disturbance
miscarriage	loss of foetus usually between the 12th and 18th week of pregnancy
naturopathy	a system of medicine based on the belief that disease results from accumulation of toxins in the body, and that symptoms are the result of the body's attempts to rid itself of these toxins
oedema	water retention and consequent swelling just before menstruation
osteoporosis	thinning of the bones
pelvic inflammatory disease	inflammation of the womb, Fallopian tubes and ovaries
phlebitis	inflammation of a vein, often accompanied by blood clots
polyps	growths from the endometrium lining of the cervical canal
post-viral fatigue syndrome	a malfunctioning immune system with one or several consecutive viruses
premenstrual syndrome	symptoms experienced before menstruation
pubic lice	small blood-sucking insects which burrow into the skin
salpingitis	chronic inflammation of the Fallopian tubes
thrombosis	clots in the blood stream which block a vessel or travel as emboli around the circulation system and lodge elsewhere
teratogen	a substance that results in damage to a foetus
trichomoniasis	parasitic infection around the anus or vagina
ulcers	open sores in skin or mucous membrane
varicose veins	engorged veins

GLOSSARY OF HERBS

Aconite, *Aconitum napellus*
Agrimony, *Agrimonia enpatoria*
Alfalfa, *Medicago sativa*
Allspice, *Pimento officinalis*
Almond, *Amygdalus communis*
Aloe, *Aloe vera*
Angelica, *Angelica archangelica*
Anise, *Pimpinella anisum*
Aniseed, *Pimpinella anisum*
Arnica, *Arnice montana*
Arrowroot, *Maranta arundinaceae*
Artichoke, *Cynara scolymus*
Ash, *Fraxinus excelsior*
Autumn crocus, *Colchicum autumnale*

Balm, lemon, *Melissa officinalis*
Balm of Gilead, *Populus gileadensis*
Barbados Aloe or Curacao *Aloe vera*
Barley, *Hordeum distichon*
Basil, *Ocimum basilicum*
Bay Laurel, *Laurel nobilis*
Bayberry, *Myrica cerifera*
Bearberry, *Arctostaphylos ulva-ursi*
Belladonna, *Atropa belladonna*
Benzoin, *Styrax benzion*
Bergamot, *Monarda didyma*
Beth Root, *Trillium pendulum*
Betony (Wood), *Stachys betonica*
Bilberry, *Vaccinium myrtillus*
Birch, *Betula alba*
Blackberry, *see* Bramble
Black cohosh, *Cimicifuga racemosa*
Black currant, *Ribes nigrum*
Black horehound, *Ballota nigra*
Black walnut, *Juglans nigra*
Blessed thistle, *Cnicus benedictus*

Blue cohosh, *Caulophyllum thalictroides*
Blue flag, *Iris versicolor*
Blue rue, *Ruta graveolens*
Boneset, *Eupatroium perfoliatum*
Brooklime, *Veronica beccabunga*
Borage, *Borago officinalis*
Bramble, *Rubus fructicosus*
Broom, *Cytisus scoparius*
Buchu, *Barosma betulina*
Buckwheat, *Fagopyrum esculentum*
Buckthorn, *Rhamnus cathartica*
Burdock, *Arctium lappe*
Butter Nut *Juglans cinerea*
Butterbur, *Petasites vulgaris*
Buttercup, *Ranunculus bulbosus*
Bryony (white), *Byronia dioica*

Calamus, *Acorus calumus*
Camphor, *Cinnamonum camphora*
Cape Aloes, *Aloe ferox*
Castor oil plant, *Ricinus communis*
Caraway, *Carum carvi cardamon*
Carrot (Wild), *Daucus corote*
Cascara sagrada, *Rhamnus purshianus*
Castor oil, *Ricinus communis*
Catnip, *Nepeta cataria*
Cayenne, *Capsicum minimum*
Celandine (greater), *Chelidonium majus*
Celery, *Apium graveolens*
Centuary *Centaurium erythraea*
Chamomile (common), *Matricaria chamomilla*
Chamomile (German), *Anthemis nobills*
Chaparral, *Larrea divaricate cav*
Chaste Tree *Agnus castus*
Chestnut (horse), *Aesculus hippocastanum*
Chevril, *Anthriscus cerefolium*
Chickweed, *Stellaria media*
Chicory, *Cichorium intybus*
Chinese angelica trees, *Aralia stipulata*
Chive, *Allum scloanoprasum*
Cicely (Sweet), *Myrrhis odorate*
Cinnamon, *Cinnamonum zeylanicum*
Clary sage, *Salvia horminoides*
Cleavers, *Gallum aparine*

Clove, *Eugenia caryophyllata*
Clover (red), *TGrifolium pratense*
Cola Nut *Cola vera*
Coltsfoot, *Tussilaga farfare*
Comfrey, *Symphytum officinale*
Cornflower, *Centaurea cyanus*
Cornsilk, *Zea mays*
Couch grass, *Agropyrum repens*
Cowslip, *Primula veris*
Cramp bark, *Viburnum opulus*
Cranberry, *Vaccinum macrocarpon*
Cucumber, *Cucumis sativa*
Cudweed marsh, *Ghaphalium uliginosum*
Currant (red), *Ribes rubrum*

Daisy, *Bellis perennis*
Damiana, *Damiana aphrodisiaca*
Dandelion, *Taraxacum officinale*
Devil's Claw *Herpagophytum procumbens*
Dill, *Anethum graveolens*
Dock (yellow), *Rumex, crispus*
Dong Quai *Angelica senensis*
Dulse, *Fucus vesiculosis*

Eagle Vine *Marsdenia condurango*
Echinacea, *Echinacea angustifolia*
Elderberry, *Sambucus nigra*
Elecampagne, *Inula relenlum*
Elm (slippery), *Ulmus fulva*
Eucalyptus, *Eucalyptus globulus*
Evening Primrose, *Oenothera biennis*
Eyebright, *Euphrasia officinalis*

False Unicorn *Chamaelirium luteum*
Fennel, *Foeniculum vulgare*
Fenugreek, *Trigonella foenum-graecum*
Feverfew, *Chrysanthemum parthenium*
Figwort (knotted), *Scrophularia nodosa*
Flax, *Linum usitatissimum*
Foxglove, *Digitalis purpurea*
Fringe tree *Chionanthus virginicus*
Fumitory, *Fumaria officinalis*

Garlic, *Allium sativum*
Gentlan, *Gentiana*
Gentian (yellow), *Gentiana lutca*
Geranium, *Geranium maculatum*
Ginger (Root), *Zingiber officinale*
Ginseng:
   Asiatic, *Panax ginseng*
   Siberian, *Eleutherococcus senticosus*
Goat's rue, *Galega officinalis*
Golden Rod *Solidago virgaurea*
Goldenseal, *Hydrastis canadensis*
Gotu Kola, *Hydrocotyle asiatica*
Grape root (Oregon), *Berberis aquifolium*
Gravel root, *Eupatorium purpureum*
Greater celandine, *Chelidonium majus*
Grindella, *Grindelia camporium, Grindelia cuneifolla, Grindelia squarrose*
Groundsel, *Senicio viscosus*
Gypsy weed (Bugie Weed) *Lycopus europaeus*

Hawthorn, *Crataegus monogyna*
Heartsease, *Viola tricolor*
Heather, *Calluna vulgaris*
Hibiscus (red), *Rosa-Sinensis*
Hellebore (faise), *Adonis autumnalls*
Hemlock, *Conium maculatum*
Henna, *Lawsonia alba*
Holly, *illex aquifolium*
Holy thistle, *Silybum marianum*
Honeysuckle, *Lonicera caprifollum*
Hops, *Humulus lupulus*
Horehound, *Marrubium vulgare*
Horse Radish, *Cochlearia armoracle*
Horsetail, *Equisetum arvense*
Houseleek, *Sempervivum tectorum*
Hydrangea (root), *Hydrangea arborescens*
Hyssop, *Hyssopus officinalis*

Icelandic Moss *Cetraria islandica*
Ipecac, *Cephaelis ipecacuanha*
Iris, *Iris versicolor*
Irish Moss *Chondrus crispus*
Ivy (ground), *Glechoma hederacea*

Jasmine (general), *Jasminum*
Juniper, *Juniperus communis*

Kava Kava, *Piper methysticum*
Kelp, *Fucus vesiculosus*
Korean ginseng, *Ponax ginseng*

Lady's Mantle, *Alchamilla vulgaris*
Lady's Slipper, *Cypripedium pubescens*
Lavender, *Lavandula officinalis*
Cotton Lavender, *Chamaecy parissum*
English Lavender, *Lavandula vera*
Lemon, *Cutrus limonum*
Lemon balm, *Melissa officinalis*
Lettuce, *Lactuce virosa*
Lilly (White Water), *Nymphaea odorata*
Lime, *Citrus acida*
Linseed (flax), *Linum usitatissimum*
Liquorice, *Glycyrrhiza glabra*
Lobelia, *Lobelia inflata*
Loosestrife (purple), *Lythrum salicaria*
Lovage, *Levisticum officinale*
Lungwort, *Sticta pulmonaria*
Lupin, *Leguminosae*

Malefern, *Dryopteris feliz-mas*
Mandrake, *Atropa mandragora*
Marigold, *Calendula officinalis*
Marjoram:
    (sweet), *Origanum marjorana*
    (wild), *Origanum vulgare*
Marshmallow, *Althea officinalis*
Meadowsweet, *Fllipendula ulmarie*
Mimosa, *Mimosa fragigolia*
Mimosa gum, *Acacia dealbata*
Mint (Spear), *Mentha viridis*
Mistletoe, *Viscum album*
Moss (Icelandic), *Cetraria islandica*
Moss (Irish), *Chondrus crispus*
Moss (Sphagnum), *Sphagnum cymbifolium*
Motherwort, *Leonurus cardiaca*
Mugworth, *Artemisia vulgaris*
Mulieln, *Verbascum thapsus*

Mustard:
  (black), *Brassica nigra*
  (white), *Brassica alba*
Myrrh, *Commiphora myrrha*

Nasturtium, *Tropaeolum majus*
Neroli (Orange), *Citrus aurantium*
Nettles, *Urticaceae*
Nutmeg, *Myristica fragrans*

Oak, *Lavercus robur*
Oats, *Avena sativa*
Olive, *Olea europaea*
Onion, *Allium cepe*
Orange:
  (bitter), *Citrus vulgaris*
  (sweet), *Citrus aurantium*
Orchard (Wild), *Orchid masculata*
Oragon Grape Root, *Berberis aqulfollum*
Origanum, *Ulgare aureum*
Orris Root, *Iris florentia*

Pansy, *Viola tricolor*
Parsley, *Petroselinum sativum*
Pasque flower, *Pulsatilla vulgaris*
Passion flower, *Anemone pusatilla*
Pan d'arco (Taheebo), *Tabenia impetiginosa*
Peach, *Prunus persica*
Pellitory of the Wall, *Parletaria officinalis*
Penny Royal, *Mentha pulegium*
Peppermint, *Mentha piperita*
Periwinkle (Greater), *Vinca major*
Pilewort, *Ranunculus ficaria*
Pine, *Pinacaes*
Plaintain, *Plantago major*
Pleurisy root, *Asclepias tuberose*
Poke root, *Phytolacca decandra*
Pomegranate, *Punica granatum*
Poppys:
  (Red), *Papaver rhoeas*
  (White), *Papaver somniferium*
Prickly ash, *Xanthoxylum americanum*
Primrose, *Primula vulgaris*
Privet, *Liqustrum vulgare*
Psyltium, *Plantago psyllium*

Pulsatilla, *Anemone pulsatilla*
Purslane:
   (green), *Portulaca oleracea*
   (golden), *Portulaca sative*

Quassia (bark), *Picraena exceisa*
Quince, *Pyrus cydonia*

Red raspberry, *Rubus idaeus*
Red Clover *Trifolium pratense*
Red Sage *Salvia officinalis*
Rest-harrow, *Ononis arvensis*
Rhubarb (Turkey), *Rheum palmatum*
Rose, *Rosecaes*
Rosehip, *Rosa canina*
Rosemary, *Rosemarinus officinalis*
Rue, *Ruta graveolens*

Sage, *Salvia officinalis*
Sandalwood (Yellow), *Santalum album*
Sassafras, *Sassafras officinale*
Savory:
   (summer), *Saturela hortensis*
   (winter), *Saturela montano*
Saw Palmetto, *Sarenoa serrulata*
Scablous, (field) *Scabiosa arvensis*
Seaweed (general), *Fucus vesiculosis*
Self-heal, *Prunella vulgaris*
Senna, *Cassia acutifolia*
Shepherd's Purse, *Capsella burse-pastoris*
Skullcap (Virquinian), *Scutellaria lateriflora*
Skunk cabbage, *Symplocar pus foctidus*
Slippery elm, *Ulmus rubra*
Soap wort, *Saponaria officinalis*
Solomon's Seal, *Polygonatium multiflorum*
Sorrel:
   (French), *Rumex scatatus*
   (garden), *Rumex acetosa*
Southernwood, *Field artemisla campestria*
Speedwell, *Common veronica officinalis*
Squaw Vine, *Mitchella repens*
Squill, *Urginea scilla*
St John's Wort, *Hypericum perforatum*
Stillingia, *Stillingia sylvatica*

Stone root, *Collinsonia canadensis*
Strawberry, *Frangaria vesca*
Sumac mooth, *Rhus glabie*
Sunflower, *Helianthus annvus*
Sweet flag, *Aconus calamus*

Tansy, *Tanacetum vulgare*
Tea tree, *Melalenca alternifolia*
Thuja, *Thuja occidentalis*
Thyme:
   (garden), *Thymus vulgaris*
   (wild), *Thymus serpyllum*
Toad flax, *Linaria vulgaris*
Tobacco, *Nicotiana tabacum*
Tormentil, *Potentilla tormentilla*
Tumeric, *Curcuma longa*

Unicorn (False), *Chamaelirlum luteum*
Unicorn (True), *Aletris farinosa*
Uva-Ursi, *Arctostaphylos ulva-ursi*

Valarian, *Valeriana officinalis*
Vervain (blue), *Verbena officianlis*
Vine (general), *Vitis vinifera*
Violet (sweet), *Viola odorata*

Watercress, *Nasturtium officinale*
Water Hemlock *Sium latifolium*
White bryony, *Bryonica alba*
Willow (white), *Salix alba*
Wild Alum *Geranium maculatum*
Wild indigo, *Baptisia tunctoria*
Wild Lettuce *Lactuca virosa*
Willow-herb (Rosebay), *Epilobium angustifollum*
Winter green, *Gaultheria procumbens*
Witch hazel, *Hamamelis virginiana*
Woodruff, *Asperula odorate*
Wormseed, *Chenopodium ambrosioda*
Wormwood (Common), *Artemisia absinthlum*

Yam (Wild), *Dioscorea villosa*
Yarrow, *Archillea millefolium*
Yellow Dock *Rumex crispus*
Yerba Santé *Eriodictyon californicum*

INDEX

insulin 149–51, 177
internal treatments 56–59
intestines 50
    flora 77, 79, 100, 140, 189
    formulations 60, 80, 90, 97, 142–4,
       152
iodine 22, 105, 123, 167
iodine-131 97
ionizer 91, 110, 171, 188, 233
iridology 75, 104, 107, 135, 157,
    200, 217
iron 3, 19, 26, 110–11, 146, 197
irritable bowel syndrome 188–9
itching 47, 63, 131, 132

jaundice 135, 164, 175
jet lag 162, 189–90
joints 46, 117, 224
juice fasting, *see* fasting
juniper berries 67

kelp 22, 91, 97, 105
kidneys 84–6, 100
    disease 7, 18, 28, 49, 121, 190–1
    flush & tonic 85
    stones 190–1
    tea 85, 191

laryngitis 51
laxatives 134, 142
lead 23, 94–5, 213
lecithin 80, 95–8, 102, 121, 164
leucocytosis, digestive 6
leukaemia 15, 73
lime tree flowers 67
lip-salve 136
liquorice 67
liver 18, 22, 80–3, 100, 128, 134–5,
    142, 175–6
    flush 80–1, 100, 127, 174
    tonic 81
liver spots 192
lobelia 67, 202, 223
longevity 1–2, 28, 29, 30
low-fat spreads 17
lungs 124, 158
lymph system 87–90, 136, 225, 238
    chronic purifier 90
    lymph gland formula 225

magnesium 28, 146, 161, 191, 197, 213
malabsorption 18, 21, 110
male corrective 182
manganese 118, 218
maple syrup 18, 59, 61
margarine 17–18, 174, 184
marijuana 223–4
massage 73, 206
    oil 116
mastitis 192
measles 25, 131–2
meat 6–9, 12, 27, 28, 37, 76, 96, 99,
    102, 115, 129, 141
meditation 38, 73, 113, 219
memory loss 20
Ménière's disease 193–4
menopause 159, 161, 194–7
menorrhagia 199–200
menstruation 161
    disorders 46, 52, 65, 111, 112,
       146, 197–200
    sanitary towels 159, 238
mental exercise 73–4
mental illness 28, 41, 112, 218
mercury 10, 11, 20, 23, 95–6, 161,
    204
migraine 172, 200–1
milk 9, 14, 27, 96, 97, 128, 207
minerals, *see* supplements
miscarriage 73, 201–2
    anti-miscarriage formula 202
miso soup 79, 204
misteltoe 67
mononucleosis 202
moon 43
morning sickness 203–4
mould allergy 118, 127
mouth ulcers 21, 51, 204
mouthwash 22
mucus 38, 91, 119, 141, 156
multiple sclerosis 204–5
mumps 25, 132–3, 183
mustard baths 49, 130, 137
myrrh tincture 44, 51, 124

nails 84
nappy rash 205
nasal sprays 137, 221
nephritis 190